How to Manage Dementia in General Practice

How to Manage Dementia in General Practice

Nicholas Clarke
Consultant in Old Age Psychiatry

Farine Clarke
Qualified GP and former Deputy Editor of Pulse newspaper and Editorial Director of GP newspaper

Denzil Edwards
Consultant in Old Age Psychiatry

WILEY Blackwell   BMJ|Books

This edition first published 2013 © 2013 by John Wiley & Sons Ltd.

BMJ Books is an imprint of BMJ Publishing Group Limited, used under licence by Blackwell Publishing which was acquired by John Wiley & Sons in February 2007. Blackwell's publishing programme has been merged with Wiley's global Scientific, Technical and Medical business to form Wiley-Blackwell.

Registered office: John Wiley & Sons, Ltd, The Atrium, Southern Gate, Chichester, West Sussex, PO19 8SQ, UK

Editorial offices: 9600 Garsington Road, Oxford, OX4 2DQ, UK
The Atrium, Southern Gate, Chichester, West Sussex, PO19 8SQ, UK
111 River Street, Hoboken, NJ 07030-5774, USA

For details of our global editorial offices, for customer services and for information about how to apply for permission to reuse the copyright material in this book please see our website at www.wiley.com/wiley-blackwell

The right of the author to be identified as the author of this work has been asserted in accordance with the UK Copyright, Designs and Patents Act 1988.

Designations used by companies to distinguish their products are often claimed as trademarks. All brand names and product names used in this book are trade names, service marks, trademarks or registered trademarks of their respective owners. The publisher is not associated with any product or vendor mentioned in this book. This publication is designed to provide accurate and authoritative information in regard to the subject matter covered. It is sold on the understanding that the publisher is not engaged in rendering professional services. If professional advice or other expert assistance is required, the services of a competent professional should be sought.

The contents of this work are intended to further general scientific research, understanding, and discussion only and are not intended and should not be relied upon as recommending or promoting a specific method, diagnosis, or treatment by physicians for any particular patient. The publisher and the author make no representations or warranties with respect to the accuracy or completeness of the contents of this work and specifically disclaim all warranties, including without limitation any implied warranties of fitness for a particular purpose. In view of ongoing research, equipment modifications, changes in governmental regulations, and the constant flow of information relating to the use of medicines, equipment, and devices, the reader is urged to review and evaluate the information provided in the package insert or instructions for each medicine, equipment, or device for, among other things, any changes in the instructions or indication of usage and for added warnings and precautions. Readers should consult with a specialist where appropriate. The fact that an organization or Website is referred to in this work as a citation and/or a potential source of further information does not mean that the author or the publisher endorses the information the organization or Website may provide or recommendations it may make. Further, readers should be aware that Internet Websites listed in this work may have changed or disappeared between when this work was written and when it is read. No warranty may be created or extended by any promotional statements for this work. Neither the publisher nor the author shall be liable for any damages arising herefrom.

Library of Congress Cataloging-in-Publication Data
Clarke, Nicholas, 1961–
    How to manage dementia in general practice / Nicholas Clarke, Farine Clarke, Denzil Edwards.
        p. ; cm.
    Includes bibliographical references and index.
    ISBN 978-1-118-35225-0 (pbk.)
    I. Clarke, Farine.   II. Edwards, Denzil, 1954–   III. Title.
    [DNLM: 1. Dementia–diagnosis.   2. Dementia–therapy.   3. Early Diagnosis.   4. General Practice. WM 220]
    RC521
    616.8'3–dc23
                                           2013014061

A catalogue record for this book is available from the British Library.

Wiley also publishes its books in a variety of electronic formats. Some content that appears in print may not be available in electronic books.

Cover design by Andy Meaden.

Set in 9.5/12 pt Minion Regular by Toppan Best-set Premedia Limited
Printed in Singapore by Ho Printing Singapore Pte Ltd

1   2013

Contents

About the authors

Dr Nicholas Clarke MBBS MD MRCPsych has been a Consultant in Old Age Psychiatry since 1996, firstly in the NHS and now in independent practice across London and the southeast of England. He primarily treats patients with dementia, which is also his area of research, and in addition manages elderly patients with depression, grief and stroke disease. A large part of his work involves counselling and guiding the families of these patients and working closely with their GPs to ensure the best possible outcomes. Dr Clarke has been involved in collaborative neurochemistry research at the Wolfson Centre for Age-Related Diseases, Guy's Campus, for the last 20 years. His MD in neuroscience, which was obtained in 1999, is in amyloid protein in human brain disease. He is widely published in leading medical journals including *The Lancet, The BMJ* and the *British Journal of Psychiatry*. Dr Clarke qualified from St. George's Hospital Medical School, London University, in 1984 and gained his MRCPsych in 1990 and his dual certification in general adult and old age psychiatry in 1996. He lives in East Sussex with his wife, son and numerous animals.

Dr Farine Clarke qualified in medicine from St George's Hospital Medical School, London University, in 1986 and completed the St Helier Hospital GP Vocational Training Scheme. In 1990 she moved into medical publishing firstly as a journalist on Pulse newspaper, where she gained sufficient experience writing and editing for GPs to become Deputy Editor. In 1997 she became Editorial Director and then Managing Director at Haymarket Medical Publishing responsible for four magazines: *GP, Medeconomics, MIMS* and *Fundholding*. During this period Farine also presented the medical news on Sky News every week as well as co-presenting a daily medical TV show 'Second Opinion'. She appeared on a number of other radio and TV programmes including Radio 4's 'Today' to report on clinical news and advances. She went on to be Managing Director of a range of specialist news stand magazines. Her first medical book, *How to Manage your GP Practice*, was published by Wiley-Blackwell in 2011.

Dr Denzil Edwards is an NHS Consultant in Old Age Psychiatry in Kent. He was an undergraduate at Charing Cross Hospital Medical School, London, and trained in psychiatry in the Bromley rotational training scheme and the Bethlem and Maudsley Hospitals in London. Dr Edwards has carried out research into treatments for resistant depressive illness, including lithium augmentation and transcranial magnetic stimulation. He is currently the consultant in a well established and experienced community mental health team for the elderly, which he helped to set up in 1996. This has a catchment elderly population of 17,000 and sees some 200 referrals a year for dementia.

GP's Foreword by Dr Neil Arnott

Dr Neil Arnott has been a GP Principal in Sevenoaks, Kent, since 1980 and an examiner of the Royal College of GPs since 1985. He is Chairman of both the Local Training Committee and the local Clinical Governance Committee.

I am very pleased to provide a foreword for this excellent and highly readable book on dementia in general practice. It is self-evident with an ageing population that the incidence of what can be a highly distressing illness, both for the individual, and, equally importantly, the families of those affected, continues to rise. It is somewhat of a Cinderella area of medicine, only relatively recently starting to receive the recognition and support it deserves. It also presents a challenge to those of us in general practice. This excellent book by authors who combine a first-class clinical specialism with ongoing research into the field can be highly recommended. It will appeal both to the younger GP starting their career, the GP in training, and the more mature practitioner who perhaps feels the newer challenges of managing these complex patients.

The book is extremely well written relying on the excellent 'learning material' of case examples that are familiar to trainers in their day-to-day supervision of registrars. Where appropriate, such as the chapter on consent and capacity, a more didactic approach helps to steer the practitioner through this potential minefield. In a similar way the chapter on drug and other therapies also gives good basic advice, whilst touching on some of the more complex areas of ongoing research. It also helps with some of the less clinically proven assumptions.

The layout and clearly defined chapters with brief summation at the end also help the reader with limited time, and perhaps a specific need or question. The chapter at the end, of commonly asked questions from GPs, gives us some excellent and practical tips.

I think it is probably true to say that this is a sadly under-represented area of medical education – although steps are being taken to change this – I know how very little, if any, formal training I received in this area of medicine.

As an examiner of the College of General Practitioners and a long-standing trainer I can also vouch for the validity of this book and its importance in helping to demystify this area of medicine.

I am sure that whoever reads this book will have a far better insight into this important and increasingly common condition, and I congratulate the authors on a significant and very useful contribution.

Dr Neil D Arnott
MBBS FRCGP
November 2012

Neuroscience Foreword by Professor Paul Francis

Professor Paul Francis PhD is Professor of Neurochemistry and Director of Brains for Dementia Research at the Wolfson Centre for Age-Related Diseases, King's College London. He has been at the forefront of dementia research since the 1970s and has published extensively in leading scientific journals, and is considered one of the world-wide experts today.

In my role as Professor of Neurochemistry at King's College London and Director of Brains for Dementia Research I have been involved in the research into dementia for over 30 years. During that period our understanding of the underlying neuroscience of diseases of the brain, both worldwide and in the UK, has increased at a phenomenal rate. In parallel to this our understanding of the possible causes, treatments and management of patients with dementia has also developed. Many doctors are aware of some of these developments, but often receive disjointed and piecemeal information, which can be difficult to assimilate into a busy practice. As such, I am increasingly asked by doctors if there is a book which translates the established and emerging research into practical applications, which they can use to improve the management of their patients with dementia. I am pleased to say that this is such a book.

From my extensive contacts with Old Age Psychiatrists I still have the sense that theirs remains a Cinderella discipline. This means that while there are many general psychiatrists who will see patients of all ages, there are still only a handful of specialists in the field who only see those over 65 on a daily basis. The expertise in dementia is, therefore, concentrated within a small group of doctors, many of whom are also involved in research. One of the authors, Dr Nicholas Clarke, did his MD in neuroscience in my laboratory at Guys and continues to collaborate with me. Dr Denzil Edwards also has considerable experience in the field of research in biological psychiatry. It is therefore vital that their knowledge is shared with others and disseminated more widely throughout the medical profession. In my discussions, particularly with medical and research colleagues, I came away with the strong sense that it is also important that everyone involved with the older adult adopts best practice. This will mean that no patient is simply labelled as 'untreatable' because they have dementia, or 'forgetful because of their age'. In the UK today, any knowledge shortfalls in dementia management and their negative impact on care, need to be addressed as a matter of priority.

As a research scientist I am committed to finding better and safer treatments for people with dementia. While some of these may be years away it is in my opinion vital that we do what we can to provide the best available care pathways for those who currently have a diagnosis of dementia. This will have significant impact and will improve the quality of life for both people with dementia and their carers. *How to Manage Dementia* is by no means a sterile medical tome and throughout each chapter the authors share the tools which they use to manage their patients. Sentences beginning 'in the authors' experience' are a frequent feature of this book, as the authors share their experience and observations with GPs in order to facilitate best practice.

GPs will recognise similarities with their own patients in many of the case histories which are used throughout the book as these are anonymised but real examples. And, if doctors read nothing else, I would advise them to read these histories. Each case brings to life many of the key features of dementia management which can be applied to a host of different patients and situations.

How to Manage Dementia covers all the key aspects of the disease, but most importantly it also offers GPs the tools to manage their patients to best effect. The text gives an organic explanation of the different types of dementia, while at the same time avoiding overwhelming detail about the molecular brain changes. At a practical level it gives GPs useful guidance on how to establish the correct diagnosis and its significance and importance to patients and families. The role of cognitive assessments in monitoring the course of the disease to ensure the correct interventions are instigated in a timely manner is also well explained. This book also helps doctors to differentiate dementia from other older adult brain diseases, including depression, which can be particularly challenging in this age group.

The chapter on dementia and memory drug treatments will be particularly useful for all doctors, as it not only explains how to select the most appropriate first-line therapy but also gives very useful advice on both the early recognition and correct intervention for specific side effects. Again it gives practical tips about how to engage carers and family members in the drug treatment process.

In my own experience working with the Alzheimer's Society and, in particular, their Research Network Volunteers, I recognise the need to dovetail medical management with a significant focus on furthering our understanding of dementia. This book explains not only the considerable support for patients and their families which the Alzheimer's Society provides but also details the role of the other charities and social services.

We all recognise the patchy nature of dementia services across the UK, which is, in part is explained by the Cinderella nature of this speciality as well as national funding issues. However this book arms GPs with the information necessary to insist that their patient priorities are met by third parties, be that a rapid assessment by the mental health services for older people team or suitable reminiscence therapy in a care home.

Finally the authors also acknowledge that GPs have limited time and a host of other pressures on that time, which is why the emphasis is on practical guidance. I envisage that everyone who reads this book will not only gain a greater understanding of the changes which take place in the older adult brain but also the wider implications for medical management of the ageing population.

Acknowledgement

The authors wish to acknowledge Martin Terrell, Partner at Thomson, Snell and Passmore Solicitors for his specialist knowledge in capacity and the Court of Protection, in Chapter 7.

Introduction

GPs are at the forefront of dementia management. They will be the first point of contact, not only for the patient, but also for concerned relatives, friends and neighbours. In addition, because GPs have the closest contacts within the community they are often the clinicians who are best placed to recognise early stages of disease.

Despite being the gatekeepers for dementia management, GPs sometimes find that ensuring that their patients receive the most appropriate treatment and support is not always straightforward. The reasons for this are multifactorial but include the fact that Old Age Psychiatry is a relatively young discipline, meaning that medical school training and postgraduate advice is less well established than it is in many other conditions. This also means that the depth of expertise in dementia is not readily available in the community. In addition, the rate, pace and stage of presentation and diagnosis are changing, as is the emphasis on available treatments. Furthermore, dementia support services are patchy and vary across the country, not least because government initiatives on dementia care seem to alter on an annual basis, but also because of the limits on resources.

This makes it difficult for GPs to always be aware of what services are available as well as how to access them. This book will explain the existing and emerging expertise on dementia diagnosis and management including the role of Admiral Nurses, community psychiatric nurses, specialist old age care managers and a new breed of managers in specialised dementia care homes, the latter of which tend to be private. It will also detail how GPs can work with the services available to decrease the pressure on their own workload while ensuring patients and their families obtain the best possible support. The authors work closely with GPs and recognise the need to

How to Manage Dementia in General Practice, First Edition. Nicholas Clarke, Farine Clarke, and Denzil Edwards.
© 2013 John Wiley & Sons Ltd. Published 2013 by John Wiley & Sons, Ltd.

provide them with a practical and clear guide to each stage in the management of a patient with dementia. As specialists in Old Age Psychiatry treating patients with dementia every day, Drs Nick Clarke and Denzil Edwards work at the front-line with patients, their families, carers and their legal deputies. They understand the issues involved and the limits on the services available but also appreciate that GPs wish to engage these to best effect. Most importantly, they know that GPs who refer patients to them and contact them for advice want concise, practical tools to deal with day-to-day patient management and also to pre-empt problems and resolve difficult issues as they arise.

Because of this, the overriding remit of this book is to provide practical and useful advice for GPs managing patients with dementia. It aims to arm GPs with the tools to manage every stage of the disease process from making a reliable diagnosis, through treatment options, to support for patients, families and carers.

Because services are inconsistent across the country many patients and families end up accessing a combination of support from the public and private sector and the book will offer a realistic account of the mixture of private and social support that may benefit patients and their carers.

Furthermore, because of the nature of the disease, the book will provide guidance on the legal aspects of dementia care including the role of the Mental Capacity Act, issues surrounding the deprivation of liberty, testamentary capacity and lasting power of attorney. Throughout the book, real GP and specialist case histories are used to illustrate important points. Personal details have been changed to protect anonymity, but the key features of these cases remain intact. In some instances the case histories may seem lengthy, and this is because dementia management often evolves as the picture changes over months and years. These authors work closely with their many GP colleagues and are aware of the limitation on their time; these cases demonstrate not only how GPs and specialists work together, but also that the degree of involvement by either doctor can vary. As with any condition which requires shared care, it is up to individual GPs to determine their own level of involvement.

The age groups affected by dementia means patients will often have coexisting and complex conditions in addition to their organic brain disease. For understandable reasons, this is an area where GPs frequently request assistance from specialists in Old Age Psychiatry and this book will help them to differentiate between conditions and also provide active management and treatment protocols.

GPs are fully aware that families and carers will often have their own strong views on Alzheimer's and other dementias and will glean information from a host of sources including the popular press, wider media and the Internet.

Some of this information may indeed be useful, but much is incorrect, unproven and potentially misleading and dangerous. This book will help GPs to deal with common queries from families and will also offer broad details on the latest relevant research so that they have an up-to-date understanding of current thinking on disease management today and in the foreseeable future.

In conclusion the authors hope that this book will give GPs a complete, practical and up-to-date overview on Alzheimer's disease and dementia, so they can manage their patients, families and carers to best effect throughout every stage of the illness.

Chapter 1 **Diagnosing dementia in general practice**

Mr Tutt was a 74-year-old man who retired after a lifelong successful career marked by his strategic abilities and intellect. Not only was he the former chairman of an international company but in his youth he had won numerous prizes for his poetry and after retirement pursued an equally successful writing career.

Some 18 months before presentation Mr Tutt drove in front of a lorry at a junction. He sustained only minor injuries but his 74-year-old wife was seriously injured. Mr Tutt was cautioned for reckless driving, and became withdrawn, although his optimistic and resilient nature prevented him from becoming depressed. His wife recovered but found it increasingly difficult to manage their busy lives.

The Tutts' professional children became concerned about their father's forgetfulness and their mother's distress and took them to their GP, Dr Smythe, who decided that Mr Tutt was not depressed, but equally wasn't his 'normal self'. In light of this and Mrs Tutt's head injury he referred the couple to an Old Age Psychiatrist.

The consultant saw them together, then separately and also interviewed the children alone. He conducted a full psychiatric history, collateral history, mental state examination, detailed clinical cognitive tests and physical examination with an emphasis on central nervous system (CNS) assessment, a CNS blood screen and MRI brain scan. Mrs Tutt had a personal previous medical and family history of depression, together with recent symptoms of early morning waking, increased tearfulness and ideas that 'life is not worth living'. Her hospital records following the accident showed considerable parietal lobe damage with intracerebral micro-haemorrhage which had resolved, albeit with residual damage, consistent with her head striking the left hand side of the vehicle. Her MRI showed residual scarring and atrophy of the left parietal lobe but with no

How to Manage Dementia in General Practice, First Edition. Nicholas Clarke, Farine Clarke, and Denzil Edwards.
© 2013 John Wiley & Sons Ltd. Published 2013 by John Wiley & Sons, Ltd.

other abnormalities, and a clinical picture which did not suggest dementia. Mr Tutt had no signs of depression but struggled with the finer points of biographical detail, for example he was unable to name some of the grandchildren he saw regularly. There were no symptoms of post-traumatic stress disorder. The consultant concluded that Mrs Tutt had a traumatic brain injury late in life, a prolonged adjustment reaction and reactive depression due to a combination of the accident, the changes in their life and the changes in her husband. This was compounded by her vulnerability to depression. She was at risk of Alzheimer's disease purely because of her history of acquired brain injury. In contrast Mr Tutt's mild concerns were more than justified because, although he scored full marks on basic testing due to his intellect, detailed testing showed changes across a wide range of functions in different lobes of his brain. This was particularly the case for recall of newly learned information. His MRI scan showed no ischaemic lesions in the white matter but some early atrophy throughout the cerebral cortex without any lobar emphasis, which with the clinical picture was consistent with Alzheimer's disease with no vascular aetiology.

This case of a married couple of similar age illustrates the difference between a brain injury with a static unchanging clinical picture afterwards, and the insidious creeping nature of dementia, in this case of Alzheimer's disease, which is typically dominated by memory loss and disorientation in the early stages and often later failure to identify familiar faces and places.

Mr and Mrs Tutt were very clear that they wanted to know the diagnoses, and a separate interview with the children confirmed this was the case. The consultant conducted a series of interviews to address the diagnosis. Mr Tutt was started on memantine with a resultant rapid and striking improvement in a range of intellectual skills. His self-confidence improved and he felt his brain was 'working better' again. He continued teaching his 10-year-old grandson about the great poets for a further 18 months during which time he made a graceful exit from his various chairmanships. Mrs Tutt was treated with antidepressants with good effect even though she had been reluctant to take them at first. The couple remained under the care of their GP and the consultant with a view to monitoring any cognitive changes in Mrs Tutt, who also received carer support for her husband's Alzheimer's disease.

How to undertake the assessment for dementia in general practice

The authors recognise that GPs have limited time to assess patients for dementia, particularly as symptoms and signs are not always obvious and may fluctuate between visits to the surgery. The following details outline best practice, and also give GPs the room to bring patients and relatives back to their surgery for further assessment and interviews, in order to build a full picture of the problem.

The right environment

As a first principle it is vital to create the right environment for the initial assessment. However well a GP knows the patient and family it's worth taking the history from the patient and the relatives separately. This is because if Alzheimer's is present, the patient will inevitably, albeit to a variable extent, give incomplete and error-strewn answers. Furthermore, in a joint interview the person giving the collateral history will often leave out important details and events in order to spare their loved one's feelings or out of 'loyalty'. All too often when they are interviewed alone, they will admit a fear of verbal recriminations typified by 'the argument in the car park' should they report things the patient is unaware of. Relatives cite outright anger and hostility, the accusation of exaggerating the problem or 'trying to put me in a home' as reasons for withholding a full history when the patient is present.

The rules governing confidentiality between doctors, patients and relatives are well known and, in principle, permission to release information is required. This permission can be implicit by the patient bringing a spouse with them, or obtained through verbal or more formal written consent. A GP can receive and hold information about a patient in any form without their consent. This is useful when asking for emails and letters relating to the patient, even if the GP is not yet 'allowed' to talk to a spouse or relative. However, if a GP acknowledges that the patient is in their care to a third party, this does breach confidentiality if there is no evidence that this party knew about the GP's involvement.

The history

The history of the presenting complaint from the patient and relative

The aim for the GP in the first instance is to listen to what the patient describes as 'complaints' and establish their order and duration, even if there doesn't appear to be any illness. Commonly the patient will be brought in and declare: '*There's nothing wrong with me*', which makes the collateral history from the spouse very important.

It is important to establish what is meant by 'memory loss' and the exact nature, density and consistency of the memory complaint. Loss of distant memories is more likely in Alzheimer's disease or another profound physical impairment of brain function. Memory loss in the recent past by which we mean 5 months to 15 years or more is also more indicative of Alzheimer's disease. Newly formed memory loss within 5 minutes to 15 hours is suspicious of Alzheimer's disease but could also be due to depression or poor concentration. Immediate memory loss within 15 seconds is suspicious of depression or poor concentration if in isolation, but may be present in rarer cases of Alzheimer's disease showing a striking impairment of immediate memory. For example a patient's daughter leaves her mother's room in a residential home and the patient turns to the nurse and says, '*Is my daughter ever going to visit?*'

The collateral history
Because of the nature of the disease there are several clues in the history about which the patient may be unaware but which the relative can clearly describe.

The most typical clue is a change in intellectual function which is commonly described as, '*I have to keep repeating myself*', '*He/She doesn't seem to pay attention*', or '*We can't talk anymore*'.

Other symptoms include 'following' behaviour, anxiety about being left alone and the inability to perform tasks which once were easy.

Unusual symptoms may include a flip or inversion of personality, for example when the vicar pinches the bottom of every female nurse, hallucinations or daytime impaired level of consciousness. The latter is different from a nap after lunch from which the patient is difficult to rouse, and indicates rarer dementias.

The previous psychiatric history
Generally this is irrelevant or contains no illness of significance. However, a history of recurrent depression or bipolar disease should raise the suspicion of depressive pseudodementia. Schizophrenia has its own pattern of cognitive deficits that are not progressive or generalised and dementia is not more common in these patients. Past admissions for unsuccessful suicide attempts and alcoholism, with the accompanying risk of brain damage and later dementia, should be taken into account.

Points in the previous medical history
A simple neurological general enquiry into diplopia, paraesthesia, focal weakness, fits, fainting episodes or incontinence may indicate occult intracranial pathology. Past brain injury from trauma, anoxia, prolonged hypoglycaemia or status epilepticus also increases the risk of dementia.

Physical diseases which may mimic or exacerbate dementia include hypothyroidism, pernicious anaemia with missed treatment, poorly managed diabetes mellitus, high blood pressure, ischaemic heart disease, tobacco-related diseases and excess alcohol consumption, either in the past or present.

Significant family history
Dementia does not typically run in families. However any multigenerational history of the disease occurring in up to 50% of family members, which presents under the age of 60, should raise the possibility of familial aetiology.

Sporadic history, as in '*my mother had dementia in her eighties*' is irrelevant to the diagnosis.

However, a family history of dementia-related conditions, such as cardio-vascular disease, may be relevant.

Relevant social history
The length of time a patient has lived in their house, the amount of help around and how close their immediate family are, are all of major importance not just in making the diagnosis but also in the prognosis and management. This is particularly true for the first two thirds, or 6–8 years, of the course of the illness. It is worth establishing who does the practical activities including shopping, cooking, laundry, and the bills and, if this used to be the patient, when and why that stopped.

Setting the personal history against the presenting complaint
Understanding the patient's premorbid intellect helps to put symptoms into the context of their ability. Their age at leaving school, academic perform-ance between the ages of 11 and 15 or 18 to include exams such as the school certificate, matriculation, O and A levels and their 'favourite' subjects together with details of their further education are all relevant. A full career history, including national service, part-time work, promotions and awards, also informs the assessment. For women who may not have had the same edu-cational opportunities, a useful assessment includes evidence of manage-ment skills in organisations such as the Women's Institute or quasi-professional roles in, for example, the Citizen's Advice Bureau or evidence of mathemati-cal ability with prizes for puzzles.

A professor of engineering who can't do *The Times* crossword as fast as he used to is reporting an objective and subjective but significant finding. In contrast, a patient who struggles to spell a five-letter word in reverse may admit they were '*never any good at spelling*' or '*missed a lot of school*', which can be shorthand for illiteracy and any test should take this into account.

The temporal gradient is a useful tool to investigate likely types of demen-tia and brain damage from the personal history. This involves looking far back into the patient's personal memory until they remember normally. For example, a patient aged 75 may not remember his final job or the celebration of a 40th wedding anniversary one decade before the interview, but will remember the places where he played golf on holiday in his fifties or earlier. As the disease progresses the memory deficit reaches further and further back into his longest surviving memories, ultimately destroying recollection of the name of his secondary school or the place where he grew up. The temporal gradient is long and shallow in Alzheimer's disease but it is steep in alcohol-related disease or brain injury.

The examination

Psychiatric examination
While conducting the psychiatric examination it is worth noting that insight is present in early dementia. This becomes eroded to varying degrees in terms of both speech and depth depending on the individual and the disease. Eventually insight is lost, although in some subtypes of frontal lobe disease it may be preserved for a relatively long period.

The psychiatric examination involves assessing the following parameters.
- **Appearance and behaviour:** is the patient dishevelled, unkempt or odorous?
- **Speech:** for loss of fluency or disruptions in grammar which might suggest semantic dementia.
- **Observed mood:** depression can complicate the differential diagnosis. Unusual anger or irritability might raise the possibility of a frontal lobe dementia.
- **Subjective mood:** the patient may not always appear depressed but will describe mood change.
- **Ideation:** secondary delusions often occur with hallucinations and also delusions of misidentification in some demented patients. *'It looks like my house but I know it isn't.'*
- **Perception:** it is worth enquiring about visual hallucinations and to note if the patient looks hallucinated.

Orientation and cognition

Cognitive tests
Cognitive testing can be carried out using a number of methods. The Mini Mental State Examination (MMSE) has moved from solely a research tool via specialist psychiatrist teams to increasing use by GPs. This and other tests are detailed in Box 1.1.

Physical examination
A full physical and neurological examination will exclude any underlying, precipitating or contributory disease and also confirm any suspicions which are raised from the history.

Box 1.1 Cognitive tests

Cognitive testing can be carried out using a number of methods.

• The Abbreviated Mental Test (Hodkinson 1972) is commonly used in general practice and in the wards of general hospitals. It serves well enough as a brief screening test.

• The Mini Mental State Examination (Folstein *et al.* 1975) is still widely used by mental health teams and to some extent by GPs, despite problems with the copyright, which does not sanction such use, unless the papers are bought from the publishers. It is validated for diagnosis but not for serial measurements, so is not ideal for monitoring the progress of patients taking a cholinesterase inhibitor, despite being enshrined in NICE guidance.

• The GPCOG (Brodaty *et al.* 2002) is increasingly used by GPs. It is a rapid and simple screening test for dementia. It is available for use on the Internet at http://www.gpcog.com.au/

• The Montreal Cognitive Assessment (MoCA) is a highly sensitive screening instrument for dementia and mild cognitive impairment (MCI) which is increasingly used in general hospitals. Test papers and instructions can be downloaded from http://www.mocatest.org

• Verbal fluency tests are a useful rapid assessment tool for frontal executive deficits. They commonly test for fluency in two categories, the phonemic and the semantic. Thus, the patient is asked to produce words beginning with, for example, P (phonemic), or names of animals (semantic), and is scored on the number of items produced in a minute. A person with normal fluency will be able to give some 30 words in three minutes in either category. A score of less than ten words in one minute in each category signals impairment. Phonemic fluency is more sensitive to frontal lobe dysfunction, and semantic fluency to temporal lobe dysfunction, but there is overlap.

• The Addenbrooke's Cognitive Examination, Revised (ACE-R) (Mioshi *et al.* 2006) is a well validated tool for assessing the severity of a dementing illness. It is commonly used by mental health teams, and less commonly by GPs, as it is relatively time consuming.

The investigations

Key basic investigations

Dementia screening includes routine bloods to exclude underlying or coexisting medical conditions which are both more common in this age group but can also aggravate or mimic dementia symptoms. Tests include full blood count (FBC), urea and electrolytes (U&Es), erythrocyte sedimentation rate

(ESR), blood glucose, lipids, liver function tests (LFTs), adjusted calcium, thyroid-stimulatng hormone (TSH), B_{12} and folate. *Treponema pallidum* haemagglutination (TPHA) may be worth doing to check for syphilis.

Special investigations
Both magnetic resonance imaging (MRI) and computed tomography (CT) brain scans will not only help to exclude space-occupying lesion and normal pressure hydrocephalus but will also demonstrate the presence of lobar or generalised atrophy.

MRI scan has a higher resolution than CT scan and can better demonstrate white matter micro-vascular infarcts which are associated with dementia. However 30–50% of patients with dementia may have a normal MRI scan while 30% of normal people over the age of 65 have deep white matter lesions.

Bilateral atrophy of the medial temporal lobe is strongly suggestive but not diagnostic of Alzheimer's disease.

There are only two instances where a high level of sensitivity and specificity has been achieved on testing. This is in extremely rare family pedigrees, numbering only 60 to 100 families of early-onset disease where serial MRI scanning can demonstrate early onset in individuals. The other is a special angled CT scan of the hippocampus coupled with cerebrospinal fluid (CSF) amyloid and tau levels. These investigations are typically carried out in specialist centres, such as the Institute of Neurology, London, and GPs will be well advised to ensure their patients avoid commercial screening services.

Typical presentations of dementia in general practice

Dementia presents in a host of different ways to GPs. As already described, the most typical presentation is a patient or relative complaining about a 'failing' memory. Rarely patients will bring themselves to the surgery but far more often a concerned relative or friend will take them to the GP.

Should a patient present alone, they will typically say, '*I don't know why I'm here doctor, there's nothing wrong with me, but my husband or wife or daughter said I should come and see you.*' Complaints such as, '*I get to the top of the stairs and then cannot remember what I went up for,*' or, '*He empties the dishwasher but puts the cutlery in the saucepan drawer,*' while seeming innocuous or even understandable considering the age of the individual, must be taken seriously. Whenever a patient or relative complains of memory loss they are right.

Box 1.2 Common presenting complaints in dementia

- **Temporal gradient pattern of memory loss**. This is faulty memory for personal events over preceding 10–20 years. A 75-year-old forgets their job before retirement, or their grandchildren, rather than events from 50 years before. Example: '*He forgot our daughter has two children, he remembers the older one aged 11 but has forgotten the 4-year-old.*'
- **Difficulty recalling newly learnt information** which is registered but forgotten within a few minutes. For example a spouse will complain: '*I told him six times he had a doctor's appointment this morning.*'
- **Agnosia**: a perceptual failure of recognition, which includes:
  - topographical agnosia; getting lost in familiar places. Patients will say: '*I knew I should know which way to drive to go down the High Street doctor, I've been there a thousand times, it's stupid but I couldn't think whether to turn left or right*';
  - prosopagnosia, also known as face blindness, which typically manifests with longstanding acquaintances rather than friends or family, for example, '*I know I should know who that man is coming towards us but what's his name dear?*';
  - Capgras syndrome is the failure to identify a familiar person. Example: '*He looks like my husband but I know he isn't, he's an impostor*'. This extends to buildings, for example, '*My mother goes out shopping but won't go through the front door and says it is not her house*';
  - a rare but interesting complaint is called delusional self-misidentification: also known as the mirror sign, this is the inability to recognise one's own face in the mirror or a photograph.
- **Dyspraxias**: difficulty with conceptual understanding of physical attributes for everyday objects and their uses. Example: '*She doesn't seem to know how to use the TV remote control anymore*', '*She has to use a recipe and weigh everything*', '*He doesn't seem to know where to put the things when he's doing the drying up. I just tell him to put them all on the table*', '*I found the camera neatly hidden between the towels at the back of the airing cupboard.*'
  - Constructional dyspraxia is a disturbance in understanding of drawn or constructed two- or three-dimensional objects. GPs can test this by asking the patient to copy a complex figure, or complete a clock face drawing.
  - Visuospatial dyspraxia is disturbance of dimensions of space and solid objects. Example: '*He tried to walk between the fence and the oak tree on the front lawn but there's only a four inch gap there. He thought he could get through.*'

- **Loss of fluency of thought** together with comprehension for the spoken and ultimately, written word. For example, a patient will complain that: '*I try to avoid party conversations now as I find it difficult to follow. By the time I say something the conversation has moved on.*'
- **Apathy** in the absence of depression or physical disorder. Example: '*He doesn't seem to do anything, he just sits there on the settee staring into space. He never used to be like that but doesn't seem to mind. I do.*'

The four main types of dementia

At a general level, dementia can be defined as an inexorable, typically global progressive disease of the brain which eventually results in significant destruction of tissue, usually throughout the organ but sometimes restricted to a unilateral or bilateral single region or lobe, which ultimately results in death.

However dementia can also be described as an aberration of one specific area of the brain which undergoes a spreading pathology. This global spread and destruction of tissue may become universal, as in the case of Alzheimer's disease, where medial temporal lobe and hippocampal atrophy occur first. Alzheimer's disease and mild cognitive impairment share this pathology in the hippocampus. Opinions vary on whether, in mild cognitive impairment, the histopathological and functional changes stay restricted to this area and are non-progressive. Usually spreading pathology in all dementias will eventually involve multiple neocortical and subcortical regions to a greater or lesser extent. In some cases this will penetrate the cerebellum and brainstem.

Patients, families, the press and some doctors refer to dementia as 'Alzheimer's disease' or 'vascular dementia'. In a nutshell, these and many other aetiologies probably overlap and together represent the discernible multiple facets of a poorly understood overarching condition or conditions, which is best described clinically by the umbrella term 'dementia'.

At a clinical level, the most useful difference for GPs is not whether the patient has Alzheimer's disease or vascular dementia, but rather, whether they have one of these two conditions or the very different fronto-temporal lobe dementia and dementia with Lewy bodies. Longstanding Parkinson's disease may have its own obvious and related dementia. Other types of dementia are rare.

Some 40% of dementia patients in Europe and the USA have an Alzheimer's disease pattern and pathology, while 40% display mixed symptoms and pathology of Alzheimer's disease and white matter cerebrovascular disease. The latter group will not show large lacunar infarcts or intracerebral haemorrhage on brain scan. A further 15% have dementia with Lewy bodies or more rarely Parkinson's disease dementia. The remaining 5% include 'all other' causes.

Alzheimer's disease

This is a slow dementia of 12–14 years' duration in which short-term memory impairment and time, place and person disorientation typically present early but insidiously spread to involve all brain functions.

As described previously, the cognitive symptoms occur early and usually include memory impairment. Initially there is a failure in storage of new items, so-called 'recent' memory. With disease progression there arises difficulty in retrieval of already stored memory, so-called recent and distant memory. A shallow temporal gradient loss with proximity and time to the onset of dementia is typical of Alzheimer's disease, as opposed to memory loss from head injury or alcohol abuse, with its steep temporal gradient.

The significance of digit span

Digit span, that is the ability to remember seven or more letters forward and five in reverse, is impaired in mid- to late-stage Alzheimer's disease and other dementias. In contrast it is relatively preserved in Korsakoff's psychosis. It is often error strewn in hysterical amnesia, for example when a patient walks into the surgery and says '*I can't remember my name.*'

False memories, the veracity of which the patient is convinced, and more unusually, frank confabulation may eventually occur, in Korsakoff's psychosis.

Speech and language symptoms

Speech and language are significantly affected as the disease progresses, early signs usually include anomia or 'nominal aphasia': the inability to name objects. This is at first only for infrequently used items but ultimately both high and low frequency used nouns are lost. Verbal ability may deteriorate further with the perseveration of words or sentences inappropriately from one answer to the next. For example: '*What month is it?*' '*March.*' '*What day of the week is it?*' '*March.*' Expressive and or receptive aphasia can occur but is more typical of cerebrovascular disease.

Impairment of comprehension of others' speech is common by late-stage disease. Finally echolalia (echoing another's word) or palilalia or mutism (inability to speak) may interfere with all speech.

Agnosias, that is the failure of recognition, and dyspraxias, failure to perform fine motor tasks, despite intact perceptual and motor function, grow more frequent with the passage of time in this disease. Topographical agnosia, or the inability to find the way, is frequently affected.

On a practical note, carers frequently complain of patients losing ability to use household appliances such as the cooker or TV, or using them inappropriately such as putting an electric kettle on a gas hob, or becoming unable to use household utensils or passing urine or faeces in the waste paper bin. A frequent precursor of failure of home care is the inability to recognise familiar faces such as a spouse. This so-called prosopagnosia makes it difficult for the carer to maintain a close emotional bond with the sufferer.

Insight is usually present in the early stages but often becomes quickly limited, not least by patients forgetting they have a memory problem. In the early stages denial may also hinder insight in susceptible individuals. In the authors' experience and as illustrated in Mr Tutt's case history, the patient's emotional reaction to the diagnosis is often disproportionately stunted compared to that of their spouse or carer.

In the final quartile the encroaching damage to motor functions, including respiratory and swallowing ability, and the resultant bronchopneumonia ends in death. Neither clinical, nor imaging or biomarker tests reliably distinguish Alzheimer's in life, but the hallmarks of microscopic brain changes are well described. These show on postmortem examination (Box 1.3).

Box 1.3 Microscopic brain changes in Alzheimer's at postmortem examination

- Amyloid protein plaque deposition in the interstitial structure.
- Misformed or 'dystrophic' brain neurones packed with abnormally processed tau protein.
- Gross loss of both specific localised neurotransmitter pathways and the global generic cortical pyramidal neurones and cortico-cortical neurones that make up the majority of the brain.

Box 1.4 Neuroimaging changes in Alzheimer's

The clinical progression of Alzheimer's disease is mirrored by positron emission tomography (PET) scanning which shows the start of the disease in the hippocampus, which is the headquarters of memory, emotion and pain integration in the brain. PET scanning shows this is followed by amyloid seeding over the front half of the brain at first which spreads backwards. In contrast, the so-called tau tangles appear first in the parietal and temporal lobes and spread from these. Eventually the effects are seen over the entire brain and nerve cells die at a rate of 3–4% per year.

Vascular dementia

Pure vascular dementia is rare. Like any other dementia it is progressive and ultimately global in its deterioration. Its various forms have been defined mainly by brain scan and are largely only of use for research purposes.

GPs see far more patients with stroke than with vascular dementia, but many of these patients will be concerned about developing Alzheimer's simply because their brains are not working as they once did. Although there is a relationship between cerebrovascular disease and dementia in some patients, it is impossible to link the extent of a stroke with the likelihood of developing progressive brain disease.

An obvious index event, such as a recoverable cortical or brainstem stroke, can also herald the early stages of the condition to both patients and their clinician. However, more typically patients will either have been unaware of the existence of past strokes for many years, or they will have apparently recovered fully from them.

Mr Morris was an 80-year-old former senior naval officer who had retired in his 50s but continued to sail competitively for fun, and was captain of his local sailing club. Post retirement he also remained actively employed managing a property portfolio.

One New Year's Eve, Mr Morris turned to his wife and asked if they should send their Christmas cards soon? She was taken aback, and realised that he could not remember anything of the large family gathering they had just had, nor vast swathes of memory for the preceding 3 weeks.

Mrs Morris immediately took her husband to their GP, Dr Abel. Dr Abel suspected an acute event and referred Mr Morris to a neurologist, but by the time of the appointment most of his recall had returned and a diagnosis of transient global amnesia of vascular origin was made. The MRI scan showed no discrete lesion but moderate white matter damage with no treatable cause.

Several months later Mr Morris returned to Dr Abel with careful notes about his symptoms, and asked: 'Am I getting dementia, doctor, as my mind doesn't seem to work as fast a it used to?' Dr Abel was unable to find any defects on cognitive testing but in light of Mr Morris's clarity about his complaint referred him to a consultant Old Age Psychiatrist.

The specialist, together with a professor in clinical psychology, conducted full psychometric tests which revealed little other than anxiety at this stage. However they asked to review Mr Morris over the coming months.

During this period he became increasingly irritable and preoccupied and was prescribed a selective serotonin re-uptake inhibitor (SSRI) to treat atypical depression, which produced significant improvement in his mood, irritability and sense of distress about his reported shortcoming.

Over the next 3 years Mr Morris continued to report the shortcomings in his ability, he continued to be assessed by his GP and specialists but showed no signs of deterioration.

After 2 years the SSRIs were stopped, but symptoms returned within a year, this time with mild alterations in cognitive function. Both were immediately restored by restarting the antidepressants.

By year five Mr Morris' careful notes about his complaints were exactly the same as at his first presentation, although he felt there had been an insidious and consistent deterioration.

However, Mrs Morris, their daughter and GP agreed he had become less flexible, astute and confident in dealing with his financial affairs. At the same time his cognitive tests dropped below their usual maximum possible scores in some areas. One particular test into 'executive' function fell by 10% but still remained twice the national average.

Scans continued to show moderate white matter damage.

In light of the step down in ability, the possibility of a progressive illness was acknowledged and Mr Morris was started on a trial of an anticholinesterase. Within weeks he returned to his previous high scores of maximum function on cognitive testing but continued to feel he had lost some ability.

Eighteen months later, Mr Morris threw a table lamp towards his young grandchild. This uncharacteristic behaviour marked another step reduction in function.

This case illustrates some of the most typical features of vascular dementia: a sudden onset of cognitive decline over a period of days or weeks followed by several plateaux of extended stable function from weeks to years, typically interspersed with sudden step-like periods of deterioration. This is set against background evidence of cerebrovascular pathology, in this case of white matter change.

Step-like deterioration

Step-like deterioration is one of the most interesting features in this disease. A deterioration or 'step' is typically described by a patient as:

- a difficult to understand sense of malaise;
- a brief self-limiting loss of functions of the brain region most affected, such as a transient ischaemic attack involving the middle cerebral artery territory in the motor cortex; or
- occasionally the total loss of recall for a swathe of memory most likely to be of recent origin in a transient global amnesia.

Relatives will typically describe the following:

- '*They're much worse*';
- '*He's been confused since last Monday*';
- '*Last week she suddenly started going down the drive, shouting at a tree. She said she could see an Alsatian in it. She's not doing it now, but she's not herself.*'

This step reduction in performance typically takes a matter of minutes or hours, reaches its nadir and then slowly begins to recover over a period of days or weeks. After a further few weeks, the relative may say that there has been some improvement but will nearly always describe a slight downward shift in overall function, even though the acute crisis is fully resolved and the current clinical picture is stable.

GPs will often see similar patterns of deterioration with limited recovery after a range of illnesses from infections to inflammation in their elderly patients. The underlying cause of this irreversible decline in cognitive abilities is unknown but is clearly not solely due to a single ischaemic or micro-haemorrhagic brain event.

TIA may be an important marker for future dementia

Transient ischaemic attack (TIA) is defined as acute stroke-like neurological impairment that lasts for a few hours and which, by definition results in no permanent damage to brain tissue. Having said that, a TIA can be followed by an actual stroke, particularly in the first 48 hours. Doctors often make the diagnosis based only on the acute neurological symptoms, such as paralysis of one side, or of part of a limb or anaesthesia, paraesthesia, loss of sight, or dysphasia. However it is worth noting that patients with vascular dementia are often left with a much longer-lasting or permanent deterioration in memory and drive after a so-called TIA. A stroke can affect any part of the brain, including the non-motor and non-sensory areas of the temporal and frontal lobes. The permanent deficit in the domains of memory and frontal lobe function may not be so easy to detect as the standard neurological signs, and will therefore remain unreported if not actively sought. Furthermore if they are detected in patients who already have a diagnosis of vascular or other dementing illness, this new sign may be ignored and presumed to have been present all along. This error can be avoided by taking a collateral history from family or friends and referring to a previous Mini Mental State Examination scores. In these cases a score from two months earlier of 21/30 will typically drop to a lower figure such as 15/30, only to recover to near its previous level. However, when the acute brain insult has recovered as far as possible and the penumbra of damaged but not dead neurones has regained function, perhaps over a period of weeks and months, the patient will be left with a lasting defect. This is due to the permanent loss of function of the neurones at the centre of the infarct. Further recovery for up to 6 months or so occurs only if undamaged portions of the brain assume the functions of the permanently damaged part.

Dementia with Lewy bodies and Parkinson's disease dementia

Dr Jones looked after 83-year-old Mrs Hewitt until she died from pneumonia but knew her 86-year-old husband would find life difficult because they had been inseparable since they met in their early twenties. He was called by the manager of the residential home soon after the funeral because Mr Hewitt insisted his wife was in the cellar and that he had seen her in the corridors. At the same time he agreed that it couldn't be her because he knew she was dead. He also complained about spots on the kitchen counter which the care manager could not see. After checking for physical illness, Dr Jones decided Mr Hewitt was grief stricken. He prescribed benzodiazepines and was considering grief counselling, but Mr Hewitt's distress worsened so he requested an opinion from the Old Age Psychiatrist.

After excluding underlying causes, the specialist who was struck by the intensity of the grief, the endless searching for a lost partner and the pseudo-hallucinations concluded that Mr Hewitt had a pathological grief reaction together with paranoid ideas, although they did not completely meet the criteria for delusions.

He began a 6-month period of grief counselling during which Mr Hewitt talked intensely about every aspect of his relationship with his wife. At the same time a very low dose of the atypical antipsychotic drug quetiapine was prescribed to temper the paranoia. After 2 months, Mr Hewitt started crying in his session but said he felt much better and that everything made sense and he could see that he'd imagined his wife was downstairs. Although he could still see the spots in the kitchen he stopped worrying about how they got there.

Over the next 6 months the antipsychotic was tailed off, and throughout this period his cognitive scores remained intact.

Two years later Dr Jones was called again because Mr Hewitt had been found wandering and confused in the town at 2 am without any shoes. An underlying urinary tract infection (UTI) was diagnosed and treated with good result.

Six months later after Dr Jones was called again because Mr Hewitt could see lights moving around in his flat; he referred him back to the Old Age Psychiatrist.

This time cognitive testing was abnormal and a provisional diagnosis of dementia with Lewy bodies was made. Mr Hewitt was started on galantamine but developed diarrhoea so was switched to donepezil. This restored Mr Hewitt's cognitive function but did not alter his visual hallucinations.

Two years later the psychiatrist was conducting a 6-month follow up when the live-in carer reported a fall when Mr Hewitt looked up to shut his curtains. Given the parkinsonian nature of this fall, namely the vertical Romberg's sign or inability to recover balance when leaning backwards, he conducted a full examination which revealed mild cogwheel rigidity and positive glabellar tap. A diagnosis of dementia with Lewy bodies was confirmed, with the onset of parkinsonism after 2 years.

Dr Jones and the specialist agreed to a trial of low-dose Sinemet which returned Mr Hewitt to full mobility together with an increase in confidence without worsening hallucinations. Symptoms of rapid eye movement (REM) sleep disorder including vivid dreams and disturbed nights settled with a hypnotic.

Eight years later Mr Hewitt continued to enjoy a high quality of life at home with a live-in carer, under the supervision of his GP and Old Age Psychiatrist.

Currently the majority of patients GPs see with dementia will have Alzheimer's disease or a mixed aetiology vascular dementia. However there is a significant minority of patients who will have Lewy body disease. This represents a spectrum of disorders of uncertain aetiology but which is identified by regional or generalised brain Lewy bodies at postmortem. The relevant ones for GPs are dementia with Lewy bodies (DLB), with a 1% total prevalence over the age of 65, and Parkinson's disease dementia (PDD) with a 0.5% total prevalence over the same age.

As is illustrated by the case above, the features of dementia with Lewy bodies are:

- fluctuating cognitive impairment which becomes consistent;
- visual hallucinosis often with secondary paranoid delusions;
- variable fluctuations in conscious level during the daytime which presents with a carer complaining that the patient is difficult to rouse;
- memory problems which are less evident at the start of the illness than in Alzheimer's disease;
- 50% of cases will have minor symptoms of parkinsonism at presentation, but nearly all go on to develop extrapyramidal symptoms, the commonest being bradykinesia and stiffness;
- there is increasing evidence of a link between REM sleep behaviour disorder, the acting out of dreams often with violent results, and dementia with Lewy bodies;
- increased sensitivity to the adverse effects of neuroleptic antipsychotic drugs which far exceeds that seen in other dementias – they will exhibit extreme parkinsonian side effects together with dramatic confusion and general deterioration to the point of near-absolute contra-indication of this drug group.

Parkinson's disease dementia

Parkinson's disease dementia occurs at least 1 year after presentation with one of the typical Parkinson's disease motor syndromes. In reality only 50% of patients will have dementia after one decade and 83% after two. Apart from this timing difference, once it emerges, the features of both dementias are broadly similar.

Fronto-temporal lobe dementia (FTLD)

Mr Jones was a 65-year-old previously fit and active self-employed engineer who was taken to his GP, Dr George, by his wife who complained that he 'wasn't himself'. Mrs Jones said that her husband seemed to 'lack purpose and initiative', which was out of character for him. Two months previously in an 'odd' incident he had fallen and knocked himself out on the pavement after his usual two glasses of rosé in the pub. He thought he had tripped on a badly maintained paving stone. He was admitted to hospital for investigations including a CT brain scan, which revealed no abnormalities, and was discharged after 24 hours.

Dr George knew Mr Jones well and had successfully treated him for one episode of depression 5 years previously. A detailed history and examination including an assessment using Beck's depression scale, found a score of 18/63 indicating mild depression. Dr George prescribed escitalopram, but because Mrs Jones was very clear that this episode was 'different' from last time he also referred him to a psychiatrist. This specialist thought there was an organic flavour to the symptoms and requested a further review by an Old Age Psychiatrist.

On more subtle questioning this specialist found Mr Jones displayed 'inappropriate schoolboy humour' which was inconsistent with his premorbid personality. His time orientation and short-term memory were scarcely impaired but were not perfect, scoring 27/30 on Mini Mental State. He also had a surprising amount of retrograde and anterograde amnesia from his head injury despite the lack of any obvious significant brain damage.

There was no consistent evidence of depression although Mr Jones was demoralised that he had wound up his lucrative and demanding small engineering firm 6 months before. He described drinking three bottles of whisky a week after work with his two close partners in his forties and fifties, but never experienced withdrawal or dependence. His wife confirmed he drank little more than one or two glasses of wine a day for the previous 15 years.

All other detailed clinical cognitive tests of lobar function fell within the normal or above average range. Physical examination and central nervous system (CNS) blood screen revealed no signs of alcohol abuse or liver disease.

CNS examination was normal, including the absence of any frontal signs. A subsequent MRI brain scan showed mild bilateral cortical atrophy involving the frontal and anterior temporal lobes with little else except very mild deep white matter cerebrovascular hyperintensities, consistent with a man of his age.

A diagnosis of likely fronto-temporal lobe dementia was made, Mr Jones was commenced on a cautious trial of low-dose donepezil in addition to the antidepressant and referred to a teaching hospital neurology centre. Whilst awaiting that appointment, Mr Jones went to Dr George complaining of difficulty swallowing and speaking.

An urgent barium swallow was done to exclude a physical obstruction. The Old Age Psychiatrist also reviewed him urgently and found he lacked concern about his symptoms. The muscles of his left thenar eminence twitched while his hand rested on the desk and his wife confirmed this had been affecting him for a few days and had put it down to nervousness. This time full physical examination showed widespread fasciculation of the large and small voluntary muscle groups across the torso and limbs with clonus and increased spinal reflexes in the lower limbs. An urgent consultant neurologist review confirmed this and noted likely early muscle wasting of the deltoids and quadriceps. Electromyographic (EMG) testing of muscle and spinal nerve function showed typical changes of amyotrophic lateral sclerosis. A provisional diagnosis of motor neurone disease complicating fronto-temporal lobe dementia was made and Mr Jones was referred to a national centre.

This case illustrates some of the key findings in fronto-temporal lobe dementia, which typically occurs in younger adults, ranging from 45 to their mid 60s. As the name suggests the condition affects only the frontal lobes or temporal lobes either unilaterally or bilaterally, even into the terminal stages of the condition.

It is an aggressive and rapidly developing dementia, destroying 6% of brain tissue per year compared to 3% in Alzheimer's disease.

The variants include:
- frontal type, which is typified by loss of judgement and defects in reasoning;
- semantic type, with loss of language skills. This group includes Pick's disease.

Unlike in Alzheimer's disease, patients will show considerable preservation of orientation, memory, and the ability to understand words and use objects in the world around them late into the disease. However they do demonstrate marked behaviour, personality change or exaggeration, disinhibition, apathy, speech impairment and stereotypic movements such as pursing the lips to

Box 1.5 Features of fronto-temporal lobe dementia

In the early stages the patients may exhibit a variety of symptoms:
- disinhibition: to include offensive language and/or offensive attitudes;
- lack of judgement in social situations which can include a lack of their usual sympathy or care for other people's feelings; at work they may make unwise or overconfident decisions or overreach in their business in financial matters;
- apathy and lack of motivation which can be prominent early signs which may lead to the misdiagnosis of depression.

sip an invisible cup and sometimes parkinsonism, usually with an abnormal electroencephalogram.

Some 10% of all fronto-temporal lobe dementias are marked by the emergence of motor neurone disease.

Early diagnosis is vital

Early diagnosis is vital as the social consequences of this disease can be devastating. Patients at this age will be working or have dependent children and be expected to behave like healthy and responsible adults in a range of social situations. As the condition and their behaviour worsens, they will be subject to increasing difficulties. They may be repeatedly reprimanded at work, eventually losing their jobs, or if they own a business will find both staff and customers questioning their actions and drifting away.

Early diagnosis will not only help to mitigate the inevitable emotional stresses at home and at work and but can also make a financial difference. This is because once family, friends and employers understand the reasons for the patient's behaviour they are less likely to treat them punitively. Furthermore, although employers may still find inappropriate behaviour and poor performance unacceptable, they may be more sympathetic and provide a softer landing and gentler options. For example the patient may be retired on medical grounds with its associated benefits rather than undergoing a harsh disciplinary procedure resulting in summary dismissal.

Families and employers who are prepared may be able to avoid any social, financial or legal consequences of a patient's inappropriate actions as a result from their illness.

Overall, early diagnosis gives everyone involved more time to prepare in physical, financial, structural and emotional terms for the future.

Key points

- Dementia is inexorable progressive brain disease resulting in loss of up to 50% of brain tissue.
- A patient complaining of memory loss, however elderly, is probably right.
- Obtaining a collateral history from a reliable source is vital.
- The Temporal Gradient, Specific Naming, FAS, and GPCOG are useful cognitive tests for GPs,
- Patients with dementia can have normal MRI scans.
- Alzheimer's disease and vascular dementia should be differentiated from Lewy body and fronto-temporal lobe dementia.
- Step-like deterioration is a key feature of vascular dementia.
- 10% of patients with fronto-temporal lobe dementia will develop motor neurone disease.
- Parkinson's disease dementia occurs at least 1 year after presentation with parkinsonian symptoms.
- Early diagnosis of fronto-temporal lobe dementia can make a financial, legal and emotional difference to patients and their families.

References

Brodaty, H., Pond, D., Kemp, N.M. *et al.* (2002) The GPCOG: a new screening test for dementia designed for general practice. *Journal of the American Geriatrics Society*, **50(3)**, 530–534.

Folstein, M.F., Folstein, S.E. & McHugh, P.R. (1975) 'Mini-mental state'. A practical method for grading the cognitive state of patients for the clinician. *Journal of Psychiatric Research*, **12(3)**, 189–198.

Hodkinson, H.M. (1972) Evaluation of a mental test score for assessment of mental impairment in the elderly. *Age and Ageing*, **1(4)**, 233–238.

Mioshi, E., Dawson, K., Mitchell, J., Arnold, R. & Hodges, J.R. (2006) The Addenbrooke's Cognitive Examination Revised (ACE-R): a brief cognitive test battery for dementia screening. *International Journal of Geriatric Psychiatry*, **21(11)**, 1078–1085.

Chapter 2 **Complex pictures of dementia**

For those GPs who have been managing a patient with a pre-existing condition for many years, the onset of dementia can result in a complex picture which requires a new approach to overall treatment. Similarly there are a number of conditions which may be misdiagnosed as dementia. This chapter divides into dementia where it coexists with physical disease, including diabetes and chronic obstructive airways disease, and where it coexists with psychological conditions such as depression, grief and anxiety. It also highlights the relevance of conditions which cause pain in dementia. The chapter will also discuss how to ensure patients who develop dementia continue to comply with their medication for a pre-existing condition throughout the course of the disease.

Dementia and physical disease

Dementia and diabetes

GPs will know that the ideal care in diabetes involves joint management with a patient who is often highly informed and understands the importance of diet and self-monitoring, the types of insulin formulation and the need to keep appointments with specialists such as ophthalmologists. In patients with dementia GPs should prepare themselves to eventually be at the other end of the care spectrum in diabetes. By this we mean their main aim will be to avoid hypoglycaemia and the worst excesses of high blood sugars, rather than focus on prevention of long-term complications such as weight gain, retinopathy and renal disease.

This cultural shift in thinking about diabetes may cause discomfort, but the reality is that as the patient's dementia progresses, the emphasis of the

How to Manage Dementia in General Practice, First Edition. Nicholas Clarke, Farine Clarke, and Denzil Edwards.
© 2013 John Wiley & Sons Ltd. Published 2013 by John Wiley & Sons, Ltd.

diabetes care needs to adjust in parallel, with an eye always on what is appropriate and safe.

For those patients with established diabetes, changes in blood glucose levels can affect their dementia symptoms, although distinguishing which changes are due to the dementia and which to the worsening diabetic control can be difficult. At a practical level it does not really matter as long as the glucose is bought back within normal limits at which point the symptoms will improve.

A patient with diabetes in early life, when the focus is on preventing medium- and long-term complications, who develops dementia in later life will experience key shifts by the fourth or fifth year of the disease. These shifts will impact the ability to maintain a preventative approach as well as the need for it. Typically the patient's understanding and pattern of eating will alter, often accompanied by an increase in carbohydrate intake. They will stop understanding the importance of blood testing and may be frightened by regular finger pricks done by a third party. They will also fail to understand the need for eye checks, and may fail to attend appointments or to comply with instructions during retinal examination.

Also by this stage the patient may only have a few years of life remaining, meaning the GP will have to balance the needs and desires of the individual against the resources available and the value of long-term aims in management.

Other acute complications which are worth focusing on in patients with dementia and diabetes include urinary tract infection, oral and vaginal candidiasis, cellulitis, and intertrigo and ulcers, the latter two of which may also be accompanied by secondary bacterial infection.

Once the means of prevention of acute disturbance in patients with diabetes and dementia are agreed, their day-to-day management requires review with the spouse, district nurses and mental health service team. In the early stages of dementia and when the patient is living at home, a spouse may take on diabetes care but this depends on their own age and personal resources. Therefore the team needs to discuss and agree all elements of care, including the number of injections, the number of finger pricks for blood glucose and the number of visits to or by third parties to oversee prevention of diabetic foot pathology and eye complications. This means management will be appropriate for the patient. It may be further reviewed as dementia progresses.

It could be argued that when the patient loses mobility and is no longer able to, for example, attend the ophthalmology clinic, the GP is best placed to oversee specialist care. Unfortunately at the time of writing, specialist dementia care in disciplines such as ophthalmology is not a key focus for the NHS.

In conclusion, the overall aim is to manage patients with diabetes and dementia as the GP would any other patient with diabetes, i.e. to keep them at the 'actively treated' end of the spectrum for the first few years of their period of dementia. However GPs need to be sensitive to the need to shift them to the lower end of the spectrum in the later years of their disease. Clearly every patient is different and the change will occur at different stages but overall the process will take between 5 and 10 years. In the later stages, the district nurse will typically give fewer injections of different insulin formulations, conduct less frequent routine blood glucose measurements and run the patient at a slightly higher than ideal blood glucose level.

A diagnostic marker
Finally, if a patient with historically well controlled diabetes presents with unexpected poor control it is always worth considering early dementia in the differential diagnosis. The patient may have lost their ability to manage the disease, as well as the ability to recognise factors such as early warning signals for hypoglycaemia.

Dementia and cardiovascular disease
There is a well recognised aetiological link between cardiovascular disease and the later development of dementia. The preventative measures are discussed elsewhere in this book. This section focuses on the management interrelationship between the two conditions where they coexist.

Management of hypertension remains relatively straightforward in patients with dementia provided they take their medication and are properly monitored. It is worth noting here that a wide range of psychotropic drugs can cause postural hypotension and thus patients already on antihypertensives may be primed to experience sudden problems even if the postural effect from a new psychotropic drug is small.

Another area of pathological synergy is between these drugs and the idiopathic postural hypotension seen as part of parkinsonism. Clearly, managing these patients is challenging and requires specialist input. Each drug requires adjustment in turn and usually the psychotropics are withdrawn first. On the whole, dementia memory drugs are not major culprits in this area. However, the clinical situation may not always permit withdrawal of psychotropics as the case history below illustrates.

Mrs Simon was a 72-year-old woman on long-term antihypertensive therapy, managed by her GP, Dr True. When her husband of 50 years died, she suffered an acute grief reaction and Dr True admitted her to a nursing home to increase her support while he oversaw her expected recovery. However when Mrs Simon developed delusional ideas that the staff were trying to poison her, he asked an Old Age Psychiatrist for a joint assessment. Together they diagnosed early dementia and prescribed an anxiolytic, with advice to staff on how to manage her ideas, neither of which produced significant benefit. However Mrs Simon did improve briefly when she was sent back to her own home, but deteriorated again after 4 weeks.

This time the psychiatrist started a low-dose antipsychotic, quetiapine 25 mg OD, which produced symptom relief for 2 months. He then started Mrs Simon on Aricept which improved her cognitive function. Mrs Simon was reluctant to stay at home alone and was moved to another nursing home where she appeared to settle. Dr True was called when she began to fall over and, in addition to postural hypotension, he also found that she had some extrapyramidal symptoms including hypersalivation and cogwheel-type rigidity of the limbs.

At this stage Dr True and the psychiatrist discussed the situation in detail with Mrs Simon's family who were very clear that the main priority should be to ensure she was not terrified. With this aim, three doctors, Dr True, the psychiatrist and a specialist Care of the Elderly Physician began to trial adjusting Mrs Simon's drugs. Throughout the process they also monitored her electrolytes, vascular tone and extrapyramidal side effects. Discontinuing the antipsychotic drug did improve the parkinsonian symptoms but the paranoid delusion returned, albeit a fear of being knifed rather than poisoned.

A trial of stopping the Aricept improved her falls slightly, perhaps by improving her cardiovascular compensation to postural hypotension, but did not alleviate the parkinsonism. Eventually Mrs Simon was maintained on a very low-dose antipsychotic, a reduced-dose antihypertensive and also a very low-dose anti-Parkinson's drug which minimised side effects while maintaining the highest quality of life.

The key points to take away from the case history above include:
- most antidepressants other than selective serotonin re-uptake inhibitors (SSRIs) carry significant risk of postural hypotension; this is particularly true of the older tricyclics which are often used at night;
- all antipsychotics carry similar risks;
- beta blockers have no place in the first-line management of hypertension or anxiety in the elderly as they carry a raft of physical and psychological side effects;
- cholinergic drugs may exacerbate first-degree heart block and cause bradycardia; this means that initiating these drugs in patients with a resting heart rate of less than 50 beats per minute should be viewed with caution and an electrocardiogram (ECG) should be performed before and after treatment;

- some anti-epileptics such as carbamazepine, used as mood agents, will have an effect on postural vascular tone, but the effect of benzodiazepines is negligible.

In terms of traditional management of cardiac disease, the increase in bypass grafts and stents means that acute ischaemia is less of a problem in this age group and nitrates tend not to be used so often. Managing cardiac failure in the elderly with dementia is similar to the approach for late stages of diabetes in dementia. The focus shifts from managing long-term illness, to treating the relapses. Clearly cardiac failure is high on the differential diagnosis for acute confusional state but GPs are usually quick to pick this up on examination.

Dementia and respiratory disease

Mr Clip was a 90-year-old, public school educated, scion of a landed West Country family. He was a fighter pilot in the war and for the last 40 years had run a successful events company. Mr Clip had four children by his first marriage, and one by the second, together with one stepchild. His second wife had died in 1990 and he remained a sociable member of the community who frequented the local pub each evening. His main pleasure was gardening and he spent most days tending his plants at home.

Mr Clip had long-standing chronic obstructive pulmonary disease (COPD) with asthma, which his GP, Dr Farish, was treating with prednisolone 5 mg daily, and salbutamol, Spiriva and Seretide inhalers. Mr Clip was good at using his inhalers when needed should his shortness of breath worsen while he gardened.

A few years earlier he was diagnosed with prostatic neoplasia which was treated with tamsulosin and bicalutamide.

At about the same time Dr Farish detected some cognitive impairment, which was intermittent at first and he was managed at home with the help of the mental health services team. Eventually Mr Clip had continuous memory loss and deteriorated to the point where he lacked the motivation to do anything, and would instead sit alone, at the most reading desultorily.

When Mr Clip told his GP that he had just been for a walk in the Malvern Hills with his mother he scored 14/30 on the Mini Mental State Examination and Dr Farish became too concerned to leave him alone. This, coupled with his increasing shortness of breath, prompted him to encourage Mr Clip to move into a nursing home.

At the home Mr Clip settled well overall however his episodes of confusion would spark a vicious cycle with his COPD: when Mr Clip was confused and forgot where he was, he became agitated, which made him severely short of breath. In the past he would have used his inhaler, however his confusion and failure to recall his disease meant he did not, which in turn worsened his short-ness of breath and also his level of agitation. At the end of these episodes, Mr Clip was exhausted.

Dr Farish asked the Old Age Psychiatrist for advice and they began Mr Clip on pregabalin 25 mg once daily, which was increased to 25 mg TDS. This drug was chosen for its effectiveness in anxiety, and unlike the equally effective ben-zodiazepines, the lack of respiratory depression side effect. Mr Clip's anxiety symptoms responded well to this treatment and he also became more confident and spontaneous overall.

This case illustrates some of the major considerations in respiratory disease in the elderly.

- When an elderly person's brain is starved of oxygen then panic, anxiety and a very disturbed mental state results very quickly. These crises may produce an apparent alteration in cognitive function and the dominant symptom is lack of attention to whatever task they are asked to perform. They may therefore be inattentive in conversation, apparently regardless of their own safety within the house and careless of their own or a spouse's drug dosages or health needs. These symptoms are also completely revers-ible at resolution of the respiratory crises. Therefore this situation merits a rapid three-way conversation between the GP, Old Age Psychiatrist and an Old Age or Respiratory Physician to resolve the problem.
- The existing behavioural and cognitive deficits in patients with dementia will be exacerbated by these crises in a similar pattern, and will also return to their previous level of impairment on resolution.
- It is possible to use drug interventions, as in Mr Clip's case.
- Psychological interventions also work, as in the case below, as long as there is a spouse or another person to support the process. The authors have increasingly seen cases where patients with COPD begin to panic dispro-portionately as they realise that their ageing spouse with early dementia is less able to provide this support during their respiratory crises.

Mr Jones was a 70-year-old man with COPD of 20 years' duration. Mrs Jones took her husband to see Dr Hans because he was 'losing his memory'. A detailed history and examination revealed clinical cognitive impairment and Dr Hans suspected his patient was suffering with the early stages of vascular dementia. He referred Mr Jones to the Old Age Psychiatrist who confirmed the diagnosis.

Over the next 5 years, Mr Jones began to present to Dr Hans with increasing frequency. Initially he would simply say he was short of breath on exertion, and

Dr Hans prescribed inhalers to control his symptoms. But eventually he became terrified simply climbing the stairs, and would panic halfway up and call his wife. By this stage Mrs Jones had also become very anxious and was afraid to leave her husband alone. She was a frail 70-year-old, and struggled to guide her husband around the house when he was in a state. The usual treatments for COPD alone failed to help and Dr Hans discussed the patient further with the Old Age Psychiatrist.

They agreed the community mental health team would help the couple. After careful domiciliary- based assessment, during which Mrs Jones said she wanted only minimal help, they found the best way to manage Mr Jones was through explanation and reassurance of his symptoms. In addition they taught the Jones to nip episodes of agitation in the bud, by using redirection and distraction techniques. For example Mr Jones learnt to stay focused on the reason for going up the stairs, rather than the climb itself, and Mrs Jones was encouraged to sit him down if he stopped halfway, and distract him with a cup of tea and a chat before attempting them again when he was calm.

At the same time they agreed with Mrs Jones that should her husband become stuck and his shortness of breath intolerable, she could call the community psychiatric nurse for an urgent assessment within the hour, before also calling Dr Hans. With this additional input, the Jones were able to manage together as a couple at home until Mr Jones died peacefully a year later.

Dementia in arthritis and pain

An important note on hip pain

One of the most important lessons when managing patients with dementia is that treating hip pain with surgical intervention, even in early stages of disease, can dramatically improve quality of life. The message is: do not withhold surgical treatment because of the dementia. Taking the patient and the team through surgery may seem potentially difficult, but GPs are well within their rights to insist that the specialist mental health services team liaises with the orthopaedic team and surgical nursing staff to manage the inevitable postoperative confusion. The irony is that these patients may end up as so-called 'bed blockers', when in reality the best management of all is rapid discharge to a familiar place, with the appropriate domiciliary support from the mental health services team. GPs can contact the team and request that their patient is seen before, during and after the surgical admission.

As with hips, knee surgery, including total knee replacement, should not be automatically excluded for a person with dementia on the grounds of their disease. This is because the relief of often severe pain and disability coupled with the relatively rapid recovery from surgery improve quality of life.

The effects of pain on behaviour in dementia

Pain may emanate from a wide variety of conditions that affect this age group, including osteoporosis, infected ulcers and neuropathy. While pain management will be the same in early stages of dementia, any pain, particularly if it cannot be expressed, is liable to cause irritability and disturbed behaviour. This is more marked in the advanced stages of dementia where aphasia or pain asymbolia occurs. This in turn increases the frustration experienced by the patient and further worsens their behaviour. Moreover because a patient is unable to explain their pain to their doctor, it is less likely to be treated.

Chronic pain with its unrelenting character and associated sleep deprivation may in turn lead to depression which will exacerbate the distress and indeed the cognitive impairment of a patient with dementia.

In advanced dementia, any pain which is made worse by handling, for example touching a sore muscle or moving an arthritic joint, may elicit a violent response towards a carer. Tragically this understandable but often misunderstood reaction can lead to a patient being inappropriately labelled as 'violent'.

Choosing the correct pain relief at each stage of dementia

In the early stage of dementia, GPs will be able to use their routine analgesic pharmacopoeia to treat pain. As the disease progresses the opiate analogues will cause increased confusion in patients. This will also be true for even the milder opiates like codeine phosphate, meaning GPs will become restricted towards paracetamol and the non-steroidal anti-inflammatory drugs (NSAIDs) if they are not contra-indicated. This approach remains true until the terminal care phase of dementia where, if the GP suspects untreated pain, it is appropriate to use opiates. This is because by this stage increased confusion is not an issue and the focus must be on keeping the patient pain free and even euphoric. It is the reverse approach to that of younger patients with untreatable cancer where there is likely to be a gradual upward titration of multiple analgesics through the illness.

In our experience the use of opiates at this later stage of dementia is often withheld completely or too slow to be started because of the fear of confusion. Needless to say they should only be administered in an appropriate terminal care setting with the involvement of family, nursing and care staff.

Dementia and psychological disease

Premorbid personality and dementia

The old axiom, dementia exacerbates pre-existing personality traits, may be true. This is another reason why it is important to enquire about the patient's premorbid personality. Behaviour that is not in line with premorbid patterns may indicate a syndrome, such as mixed depression and anxiety, which requires specific treatment. In contrast, where apparently abnormal behaviour is consistent with pre-existing traits, non-drug methods of management are more appropriate.

Knowledge of the patient's early childhood and occupational history may give clues to causes of abnormal behaviour.

Mr Finch was a 72-year-old patient with Alzheimer's disease who would repeatedly pile up furniture in the centre of the lounge of his care home, much to the annoyance of the other residents. When his daughter came to visit she explained that her father used to be a painter and decorator and this was how he began any job. Armed with this information, the staff were able to reassure Mr Finch that he had finished decorating the room, at which point he would relax. Granted, he had to be told this repeatedly, but at least the staff could manage Mr Finch with greater understanding.

For some patients traumatic events in their past will also influence their behaviour.

Mr Chase was a 79-year-old man with dementia who had lived with his wife at home until she could no longer manage, when he moved into a care home. Mr Chase settled in well, and was liked by the staff and residents as he was a sociable and kind character. He was also very proud and tidy and kept his room and his possessions in good order. However, after a few days the staff found that when it came to taking a shower or having a bath, Mr Chase would behave in a manner which was out of character, panic and refuse.

His GP, Dr Browne, had a confidential chat with Mrs Chase about her husband's refusal to bathe. With some difficulty Mrs Chase explained that her husband had told her that he had suffered sexual abuse in his childhood and although it had not appeared to affect him in his daily adult life, he clearly remembered the incidents.

Dr Browne concluded that being asked to strip in front of care staff was too traumatic for Mr Chase. He asked the care staff to take Mr Chase to the shower room but reassure him that he would be left in private to remove his clothes and wash without any chance of being interrupted. Once he understood the new arrangement Mr Chase was very happy to bathe each day.

The above example illustrates once again the need to take a careful history from the families and carers to ensure patients are treated appropriately for their behaviour. Care home staff will understand the need to be patient specific. For example they will give explicit reassurance and allow patients to go very slowly with repeated explanation, or even exchange the carer for one of a different gender.

Depressive illness with and without dementia

Depression and dementia can coexist in those aged over 65, although it is clearly important to distinguish between these two, and identify if one or both are present.

We now know that late-onset depressive illness is associated with clinically detectable cognitive alterations which might not completely reverse on treatment. In turn this has an increased probability of brain white matter ischaemic changes on MRI. However patients with mild cognitive impairment are more likely to develop coexistent depression than those with depression are to develop mild cognitive impairment. This suggests depression in dementia may have a direct aetiological link with previous mild cognitive impairment, and thus a slightly different prognosis and response to treatment.

How does late-onset depressive illness vary from that in seen younger adults?

Late-onset depressive illness has many similarities to depression in younger patients, including appetite change, poor sleep, pain, bowel disturbance, reduced energy and loss of sexual function. The latter can be significant and it would be wrong to assume that the patient had no sex life before presentation on account of their age. Hopelessness, guilt, suicidality and psychomotor slowing also occur as in the young.

However, increased appetite, weight gain, hypersomnia and low mood later in the day, akin to 'neurotic' or 'reactive' depressive illness, are rarer in the elderly than in the young. One exception is the unhappy loneliness of recently bereaved patients which takes hold in the quiet of late afternoon or evening. Depressive illness in the elderly is more likely to feature somatic complaints such as pain or fatigue, gross physical agitation and restlessness, and negative psychotic ideas. We have seen patients who assume that they are near bankrupt, their insides are blocked, that they have cancer the doctor has missed, or they are dying. Extreme cases believe that they are already dead, despite evidence to the contrary in the GP's surgery!

How do you differentiate depressive illness from dementia?

There is a number of ways of differentiating depression from dementia and one clinical shortcut is to ask the patient the full address of the surgery or their residence or care home and the date including day, month and year. The older patient with depression but intact cognition will give clear correct answers. In contrast a patient with early dementia is likely to make errors as part of an expansive reply and will give the name of the town they grew up in rather than their actual whereabouts. The severely depressed patient with psychomotor retardation may remain mute or give a simple, careless, response, such as, '*I don't know*'; and declare this repeatedly to each enquiry.

In some situations the depression is so serious that the patient appears to have severe cognitive impairment and is initially misdiagnosed with dementia. These patients with so-called 'depressive pseudodementia' usually require specialist psychiatric assessment.

Dr Greene was called to see Mrs Major aged 82, who lived relatively independently in a converted stables next to her daughter Justine's house. One day she fell on a smooth, dry floored walk-in shower area and Justine, who witnessed the fall, picked her up immediately and was sure she had not lost consciousness. Dr Greene sent Mrs Major to the local A & E who examined her and performed a CT brain scan which showed no abnormality other than minimal deep white matter hyperintensities reported as 'normal for age', and in particular no evidence of acute ischaemic stroke.

Six months later Mrs Major fell again in the early hours and pressed her emergency alarm to reach her daughter. Again there was no obvious loss of consciousness. The on-call GP decided against any further action and suggested a routine check with Dr Greene the next day. Dr Greene took a detailed history and found nothing to suggest precipitating factors, a thorough examination also revealed no obvious abnormalities.

One morning Mrs Major announced that she had appointments for the chiropodist but when Justine took her she found the time and person were correct but the date was a day too early. A few days later exactly the same thing happened over a physiotherapist appointment. Mrs Major had correctly recorded the appointments in her diary, so Justine took her back to Dr Greene enquiring about her memory. Dr Greene referred Mrs Major to a consultant Old Age Psychiatrist with a specific aim of excluding early stage vascular or mixed aetiology Alzheimer's dementia with transient mini-strokes, in the absence of any other obvious unifying pathology. He included in the referral letter that Justine's mother-in-law had recently 'died of severe Alzheimer's' in a residential home.

When the consultant psychiatrist arrived at Justine's house he found an ambulance outside and the paramedics inside treating Mrs Major for cuts to her jaw and knees. Justine explained she had not cancelled the appointment as she felt it was important for the doctor to witness her concerns first hand. She explained that she had returned from a short shopping trip to find blood everywhere, a packet of cigarettes in the flower bed, and some evidence that her mother had tried, unsuccessfully, to clean it up.

Mrs Major told Justine that she had felt 'unwell' and 'confused' whilst going to the dustbins and turned the 'wrong way' which made her fall and hit her head. She had full recall of the event including the percussive blow to her head 'like a nut hitting the ground'. The paramedic had excluded any obvious cardio-vascular or somatic cause such as epilepsy requiring hospital admission and arranged an out-patient follow-up to check her wounds.

The Old Age Psychiatrist took a detailed collateral history from Justine. Despite a limited wartime education which ended at 16, her mother rose through the ranks of a large London department store to become a manager. She was asked to leave because she got married, at the age of 24. During the 1960s she brought her two children up in Worthing whilst her husband worked overseas and only moved in with her daughter 3 years previously. This was a reluctant move as she had many friends in Worthing, albeit increasingly frail ones. Justine said her mother had failed to make new friends and also refused offers of lifts to the local shops. Justine also thought Mrs Major had lost confidence after the second fall. She would get up for a sparing breakfast with her daughter, but would then go back to bed sometimes for half the day. Justine thought her mother's trip to the garden was her first outing of that week. The consultant wondered if she had gone out for a cigarette, as her daughter laughingly said Mrs Major would surreptitiously smoke behind the dustbins. Justine said her mother did not report low mood, tearfulness nor complain of hopelessness.

On examination, the consultant found Mrs Major was fully conscious and orientated in time and place. She grasped the consultant's name and could repeat it to him 3 minutes later. She was also able to recall the events which led to her fall, and accurately describe her injuries. She denied going outside to smoke.

However when asked if life was worth living, Mrs Major smiled and said, 'I don't see the point when you get like this.' Within a few minutes Mrs Major's sadness over the loss of her husband to a sudden stroke 40 years ago came to the fore. The loss of her friends and home despite her love for her daughter was also a clear source of unhappiness and she admitted she had lost interest in everything, even the daily newspaper which she used to love reading. Still smiling beatifically she said, 'I have never been one to cry but feel as if I would like to now. But I can't.'

After a full cognitive and mood assessment a few days later the consultant diagnosed 'smiling' depression, which is a variant presentation confined largely to the elderly. He explained that poor 'memory' and 'confusion' were secondary to a combination of depressive stupor and poor concentration, which was likely to be most evident in the early morning. The timing of Mrs Major's falls may again have been related to inattention at this time of day.

He prescribed an SSRI antidepressant and within 2 weeks Mrs Major had recovered fully. She returned to her walks and newspaper, continued to smoke *rebelliously, and confided to Dr Greene at a follow-up appointment that, 'I may have needed to have a breakdown.' She thought her daughter was 'lovely' and enjoyed living with her.*

The case above illustrates some of the key difficulties in diagnosing mood disorder in elderly patients. Dr Greene had already excluded other somatic disease, but the reported symptoms of walking less, falls, memory problems and possible intermittent confusion, might have indicated an intrinsic neurological disorder, such as Parkinson's disease, epilepsy or early dementia. Indeed the specialist thought the fall and head injury on his first visit also suggested this. Furthermore the absence of any obvious sadness, irritability or flattening of emotion, and a lack of typical biological symptoms such as anorexia, weight loss, early morning waking and low mood, meant depression was not high on the differential diagnosis.

The clues for the specialist came from the daughter's report of diurnal variation, manifest by her mother's repetitive pattern of extreme reduction in motor activity in the first half of each day.

After excluding gross cognitive impairment or acute confusion, he elicited previously undeclared depressive feelings and ideas, including a loss of pleasure and appetite for life which contrasted strongly with her apparently joyful demeanour. This core symptom of anhedonia is thought to differentiate depression from almost any other brain disorder in later life. Patients have described this inability to extract joy, in however small a measure, from food, company, distraction, friendship, pastimes and family as akin to: '*The colour draining out of a picture, like a black and white television*'. It results in uninterest and a loss of appetite for life. This makes it a vital first line of enquiry by a GP who suspects depression in an older patient, as almost every other depressive feature, including suicidal thinking, can be a facet of other brain disease or part of normal ageing. It was this factor, taken together with the diurnal variation in motor activity early in the day, that supported a diagnosis of depression in Mrs Major, rather than acute or chronic organic brain disorder.

Uncovering diurnal variation
In atypical depression where patients may even deny low mood or loss of pleasure, a variety of somatic and psychological symptoms may still vary in a cyclical way which is reminiscent of orthodox diurnal mood variation in younger adults. These include musculoskeletal shoulder and neck pain, palpitations, fatigue, dyspnoea, loss of appetite, generalised free-floating anxiety, panic attacks, agitation, grief and even reported dysmnesia or confusion, all worse in the morning. Thus it is always worth asking a patient or relative

whether any repetitive variable symptom is present at or soon after waking, which gets slowly better through the day. An affirmative reply raises the index of suspicion of depressive illness, even where there is circumstantial evidence of other physical or mental disorder.

Sundowning syndrome
In Alzheimer's disease and other dementias, a specific pattern of diurnal variation occurs where a symptom such as confusion agitation, forgetfulness or mood swings gets worse as the day goes on. This is called the 'sundowning syndrome'. GPs can explore this by simply asking the relatives if it seems like the brain begins to run out of petrol towards the end of the day. Often relatives reply, with some relief, that it does.

Depression in pre-existing dementia
Classical depression can occur in the early stages of dementia and should be diagnosed and treated accordingly. Incomplete depressive syndromes can also occur and are part and parcel of the dementing process. GPs may have come across the concept of changes in mood and behaviour, the so-called, behavioural and psychological symptoms of dementia (BPSD). This is essentially a research tool aimed at establishing useful categories for postmortem brain investigation and *in vivo*, rational pharmacological treatment.

These categories include:
- affective symptoms such as anxiety and depression;
- restlessness, including agitation, wandering, over-activity and calling out;
- aggression, both verbal and physical;
- psychotic symptoms, including delusions and hallucinations.

Treating depression in dementia
Managing dementia and depression necessitates a multifaceted approach which requires that doctors and carers address a variety of physical and emotional aspects of the patient's life, which, if ignored, can worsen symptoms and increase distress at any stage.

In patients where the two conditions coexist or where the exact diagnosis is still in doubt, experience shows that drugs are effective and a trial of anti-depressant drug therapy is therefore appropriate. There is some research evidence to suggest that depression in dementia is unresponsive to conventional antidepressant therapy and is self-limiting, but the evidence base for the effectiveness or otherwise of antidepressants in patients with depression in dementia is still relatively poor, and the authors recommend a trial of treatment.

Drug choice and order of use is the same as treating late-onset depressive illness. First-line treatment is with a low-dose SSRI titrated slowly at 4–6-

week intervals to minimise side effects. GPs should bear in mind recent warnings on cardiac QT prolongation with citalopram. SSRIs can worsen anxiety in the short term. The authors have not seen any evidence of increased anger and suicidal thinking, nor the withdrawal syndromes on sudden discontinuation, which are increasingly reported in younger adults.

Mirtazapine (Zispin, Merck Sharp and Dohme, Ltd.) is a useful second-line treatment for its sedative effect in low doses in patients with insomnia, its mild anxiolytic effect and its positive effect on appetite. These useful side effects begin soon after starting treatment while awaiting the drug's true antidepressant effect.

Duloxetine may be a second- or third-line therapy. It is licensed not only for depression, but also anxiety disorder, diabetic neuropathy and stress incontinence. It is used off-licence for other forms of neuropathic pain. Like mirtazapine it has a dual antidepressant effect, increasing both noradrenergic and serotinergic transmission, which may make it a more effective antidepressant. Its 20 mg capsule preparation as Yentreve (Lilly) offers GPs the possibility of off-licence low-dose introduction before proceeding on to an antidepressant dose of 30 mg and then to 60 mg as Cymbalta (Lilly).

A third dual-action antidepressant which is effective in our experience is venlafaxine in delayed-release formulation. This drug needs to be used with caution in cases of heart disease and hypertension and requires ECG and blood pressure monitoring.

Tricyclic antidepressants should be avoided in this age group because of their anticholinergic effects. This is particularly the case if there is any degree of dementia. They may act centrally to cause memory problems, confusion and even acute reversible hallucinosis. This is in addition to the common and better known peripheral anticholinergic side effects of dry mouth, constipation, disturbance of visual accommodation and, rarely, precipitation of acute closed angle glaucoma. Their alpha-1 blockade and membrane-stabilising effects are also undesirable in the frail elderly, contributing to QT interval prolongation and severe postural hypotension.

Grief in dementia

This group of patients are at risk of bereavement during their illness by virtue of their age. Patients with Alzheimer's disease and vascular dementia often demonstrate a 'shallowing' of the effect of sad news, in terms of both the depth and duration of feeling. This is analogous to sailing on a coral sea which appears as deep as any part of the surrounding ocean on the surface, but on close testing reveals 10 feet of water rather than the 200 fathoms expected. We have observed that imparting the diagnosis at clinic often has the same impact on the dementia patient as their close companion or family at first. However on follow-up a few weeks later the patient is often relaxed or even blithe, compared to their partner who is pale, anxious and distressed. This even occurs when the patient recalls the headline content of previous discussion about their dementia. There is evidence that dementia patients require a much greater emotional association to remember a new piece of information than do healthy older people. This indicates an alteration in emotional processing. GPs can take this response into account when talking of the illness or death of a loved one to their patient with dementia. As a rule of thumb, GPs should expect the immediate impact to be as painful as for any other of their patients and exercise their usual care. However they may find the pain of the news will lessen in a shorter time than for other patients. As the dementia progresses a time may come when it is inappropriate to involve the patient in the terminal illness or death of a loved one. However this requires consideration of a number of factors, including the severity of illness, the previous relationship and wishes as reported by family and the response of the patient when the subject is gently broached. The needs of the dying partner are equally important. It is worth remembering that a patient who fails to recognise a spouse when discussed in conversation, can exhibit immediate emotional recognition when by their hospital bed.

At a funeral a patient with moderate or severe dementia will require special care and protection of their dignity and coping abilities. Families may find the prospect of the funeral with the patient present overwhelming. GPs can help by suggesting a friend or carer accompanies the patient, and brings them in and out depending on their emotional state, cognitive awareness and fatigue. They can also reassure them that the patient need only attend for part of the service. A caring companion can also facilitate a typically attenuated form of grieving by discussion with the patient in the days after the funeral. Carers report that sometimes a patient with advanced dementia will suddenly make a sad observation about the loss of a loved one weeks or months after the event, despite having failed to recognise the death at the time.

Key points

- Sundowning syndrome is a specific form of diurnal variation seen in dementia.
- The features of depression in the elderly differ markedly from the young.
- Managing diabetes in dementia requires a cultural shift in blood glucose control.
- Dementia should not be a barrier to surgical intervention in hip pain.
- Opiates should not be withheld in the terminal stages of dementia.
- GPs can give families permission to limit a patient's presence at a funeral for everyone's benefit.

Chapter 3 **Initiating, monitoring and adjusting dementia treatments**

Mr Ashley was a retired businessman who had travelled the world creating his successful manufacturing company. He enjoyed a happy family life with his wife, Victoria, and their four grown-up children, who lived locally but visited regularly with their much loved grandchildren. Mr Ashley rarely visited his GP, Dr French, but was brought into the surgery one day by his wife who said he had become hesitant in conversation and seemed to stumble over words, so that she had to fill in for him in public, or prompt him to find the right word in private. He had never been a garrulous man but was stoical and always supportive of her and the family. It seemed to her that there was also a reduction in the quality and frequency of their private marital conversations. Almost by way of incidental occurrence, she thought his memory was not quite as sharp but put this down to 'getting old', although he was only 75.

Dr French conducted a full physical examination but found no evidence of any other disease that might explain his symptoms and referred Mr Ashley to a consultant Old Age Psychiatrist for further assessment.

The specialist conducted a Mini Mental State Examination which revealed a score of 24/30 and a mild expressive dysphasia, that was symbolised by some disruption of normal syntax and structure of sentences, although Mr Ashley's understanding was intact. Of greater significance, detailed cognitive testing demonstrated that his low score reflected not only a language defect but mild loss across a wide range of lobar functions, which is typical of early dementia. Physical examination and investigations showed no distinct stroke or focal lobar atrophy, but considerable deep white matter changes. These findings led to a diagnosis of mixed Alzheimer's with cerebrovascular disease.

How to Manage Dementia in General Practice, First Edition. Nicholas Clarke, Farine Clarke, and Denzil Edwards.
© 2013 John Wiley & Sons Ltd. Published 2013 by John Wiley & Sons, Ltd.

At this time, the first licensed cholinesterase inhibitor, donepezil, had just been made available in the UK. The specialist discussed the relatively unknown benefits and risks of the drugs with Mr and Mrs Ashley who agreed to try treatment.

After 4 weeks of 5 mg donepezil as soon as Mr Ashley walked into the clinic he declared, 'I can talk again' and proceeded to demonstrate a near total improvement in his expressive speech difficulties. His other mild cognitive difficulties had also improved. This time his Mini Mental State Examination score was 29/30, the only error being a minor one relating to a date.

Mr Ashley continued donepezil at a maximum dose of 10 mg at night for nearly 5 years before his general cognition, speech and motor functions had deteriorated so that he could no longer walk long distances, or hold active conversations. Two attempts at withdrawal of donepezil showed marked immediate deterioration after 4 days which was restored by reinstating the drug. Eventually the benefits were swamped by his global physical and mental deterioration. During this time his wife cared for him at home, with a combination of support, including an employed daytime carer, assistance from the family and the emotional boost from the grandchildren after school and in the holidays. Together with Mr Ashley she attended local support group meetings and became actively involved in helping others with the disease through education.

Seven years after presentation Mrs Ashley returned to Dr French asking if it was worth trying the newly licensed drug, memantine, which was said to give benefit in advanced dementia after trials in nursing home patients. Again Dr French asked the specialist for an assessment and advice.

The specialist found Mr Ashley to have deteriorated physically as one would expect; he was at a slightly higher weight than when active and prone to feel the cold, wearing a thick coat in the warm clinic. However he also demonstrated some awareness of his condition; he was able to make eye contact, grunt appropriately or give monosyllabic answers to some questions. He was not obviously depressed or in pain. This time Mr Ashley's Mini Mental State score had fallen to 3/30, which is near the floor for this test. The specialist and Mrs Ashley had a lengthy discussion about the benefits of memantine and started a trial of 5 mg BD.

The couple returned to clinic 4 weeks later where Mrs Ashley said the little things her husband could now do made all the difference. She was delighted that he could lift his wine glass again at 6 o'clock each evening when they sat down together after she had cared for him all day. To her, this moment of intimacy was what kept her going.

Mr Ashley benefited from this drug for another 18 months and died after a 10-year illness of bronchopneumonia. His wife had managed to care for him at home throughout this period.

This case illustrates some of the key features of dementia treatment, including when to begin therapy, the benefits to both carers and patients of changing drugs when there may appear to be little hope and also how to trial drug withdrawal.

What treatments are we talking about?

Patients in the UK typically receive a cholinesterase inhibitor drug as the first line and usually the only treatment for Alzheimer's disease. All three such drugs, donepezil (Aricept, Pfizer-Esai), galantamine (Reminyl, Shire) and rivastigmine (Exelon, Novartis), act to block the effect of the deactivating enzyme acetyl cholinesterase at the synaptic clefts. This is where cholinergic neurones impinge upon the main substrate of the cortex, the glutamatergic pyramidal neurones. One drug also inhibits butyrylcholinesterase, but does not appear to exert greater clinical effect in dementia. The drugs probably act by making acetylcholine available in greater concentrations and for a longer duration in the synaptic cleft, after depolarisation of the cholinergic afferent neurone.

For UK GPs the majority of their dementia patients who are treated will receive donepezil. This group probably represents some 75% of patients. A substantial minority, around 20%, will receive galantamine, and approximately 5% receive rivastigmine. These numbers may change with time particularly as drugs come off patent.

Unfortunately, as with some other conditions, so-called postcode prescribing is a feature of dementia drug treatment, not least because of the initial overarching restrictions of NICE, as well as local budgetary restraints. To put availability in context, of all the economically developed G20 countries, France probably offers greatest opportunity for access to these drugs, followed by the US and Japan, with the UK in the bottom quartile of provision. Again this may change in time.

The situation continues to evolve, and in some areas of the UK early rates of 50% of patients being offered the drug have declined, while in others, where a negligible 5% of patients were offered the drug initially, rates have now risen.

Overall, access to treatment throughout the course of the disease has probably risen from 20% nationally, as found by the author in 2005 (Francis & Clarke 2005), but still falls woefully short of all patients being offered these drugs at some stage during their illness.

A small number of Parkinson's disease dementia patients will have been offered rivastigmine, which was licensed more recently for this disease.

The drug memantine (Ebixa, Lundbeck), which has been recently added to the UK pharmacopoeia since the onset of cholinesterase inhibitor therapy, merits special mention, not least because of its side effect profile. Memantine is an antagonist of NMDA receptors on glutamatergic to glutamate synapses of the cerebral cortex. It has been licensed both for the cognitive treatment of moderate to severe Alzheimer's disease, and behavioural disturbance of advanced dementia. It has the same dimension of benefit as cholinesterase inhibitors in early disease when used alone. When used together, a cholinesterase inhibitor and memantine combination may offer some increased synergistic benefits. Otherwise it offers an alternative first-line treatment in cases where cardiac conduction defects preclude safe use of a cholinergic drug. It is also an alternative when cholinergic drugs prove unsuccessful or cause severe adverse side effects (Francis *et al.* 2012).

Which forms of dementia are suitable for treatment?

Of the four main categories of dementia described, Alzheimer's disease is the licensed application for both the cholinesterase inhibitors and memantine. Concurrent cerebrovascular disease may complicate treatment but does not preclude it. Trials indicate the benefit of treatment outweighs the risk of cardiac complications in 'pure' Alzheimer's.

Not only can the same relevant neurochemical deficit be found in vascular dementia, but cholinesterase inhibitor treatment may also elicit clinical benefit which justifies a 3-month trial in the first instance. More often than not the exact clinical diagnosis is secondary to the pragmatic benefits of a trial of treatment.

Where dementia with Lewy bodies is concerned, the postmortem deficit of cholinergic function is even more pronounced than in Alzheimer's disease. This gave early hope that cholinergic drugs would be of most benefit in this group. In practice, however, they do not confer greater benefit than in Alzheimer's disease, although they do result in equivalent improvement. Treatment is justified in all dementia with Lewy body disease patients.

Patients with fronto-temporal lobe dementia are the exception to the inclusive approach to treatment. There is no neurochemical basis for cholinesterase inhibitor use in the disease as the cholinergic system remains relatively unaffected. Furthermore, some patients describe or are observed to show possibly worsened depression or confusion at low doses of cholinergic treatment. For these reasons, it is advisable to refer patients in this group for a trial of treatment to a specialist neurology or psychiatry clinic.

When should treatment be initiated?

Treatment can be started once the progressive and, or, generalised nature of the disease is established. As described in Chapter 1, such deterioration is identified from the clinical history through simple questioning of the patient and, more importantly, a close family member or carer. For each complaint, however long it has been going on, and sometimes this will be years, one should establish if it has got worse in the last few months or as an inexorable gradual or step-like deterioration. Doctors should also look for a widening spread of dysfunction, with an evolving pattern of different problems, which begin to spread across the domains of lobar brain function. A typical example is an early memory problem which is complemented by subsequent dyspraxias for buttoning up a cardigan or using a knife and fork at mealtimes, and topographical agnosia for knowing the way to the lavatory at home.

We have already stressed that it is only possible to establish this pattern from a reliable collateral historian who is capable of noticing, remembering and describing the changes. He or she must also be willing to acknowledge the information themselves as it is common for a spouse or child to avoid thinking the worse. They will often accept that a problem exists, but at the same time, they will step back from labelling it as progressively worse, believing this to be brutal or disloyal.

GPs can retrospectively identify deterioration through a more formal but less hands-on approach, by referring their patient to a psychologist for psychometric testing. The National Adult Reading Test (NART) will establish likely premorbid IQ and at the same examination the Wechsler Adult Intelligence Scale (WAIS III) will estimate current verbal and performance IQ. The latter will be compared with the premorbid figure. If needed, a further assessment 6 or 12 months later, will clearly establish if there is ongoing decline in performance suggestive of a degenerative process. The WAIS III in combination with other psychometric tests will also establish if there is a discrepancy between different realms of cognitive ability, that may perhaps have an anatomical locus of origin, for example a discrete worsening failure of frontal lobe executive function in fronto-temporal lobe dementia.

GPs will find using the passage of time as one of the axes of clinical investigation extremely useful in the surgery setting. By carefully documenting the findings and uncertainty of final diagnosis to date, and then reviewing these 3 months later, new developments will become apparent. Asking the family to bring the patient back should any changes occur will also help with the diagnostic process. Asking them to keep a diary of events and changes will also help families to feel they are actively managing the process rather than simply watching a decline.

GPs may find it more difficult when there appears to be a discrete but stable problem in one particular cognitive domain, a typical example being delayed recall of newly learned verbal information with or without problems of orientation in time and place. This may be definitely noticeable to the patient or others, but does not seem to be worsening after many months of reassessment at the surgery. This mild cognitive impairment is difficult to separate from early-stage Alzheimer's disease or mixed cerebrovascular dementia in the absence of other pathology. Opinions vary on the benefits of drug use at this stage, or, as importantly, the risks involved by delaying treatment. This is uncertain territory and currently involves off-licence prescribing by specialists in Old Age Psychiatry. For this reason GPs may find it beneficial to refer to a specialist prescribing clinic.

How do we monitor if treatment is working?

There is no reliable evidence regarding what might be considered a normal or expected rate of decline at any given stage of Alzheimer's disease. Despite a suggestion that the first and final quartiles of the illness are marked by more rapid deterioration, research into CSF biomarkers has not borne this out.

Generally a decline of 3–4 points a year on Mini Mental State Examination can be expected in untreated patients. The steepness of this downward curve may be similar once treated patients begin to decline. The important concept to explain to patients and their carers is that treated patients remain above the untreated curve and for this reason it is worth taking the drug. When explaining this to patients' families, the authors often use the analogy of being on a sinking ship like the Titanic: wearing a life jacket while being in the water is the equivalent of taking medication. The end result is the same, death by drowning or hypothermia, but the cognitive state of the treated person 'floats higher out of the water' than the untreated. For obvious reasons studies of the effect on end point, namely the time to death, have been near impossible. However there is evidence of delays of up to 22 months in nursing home admission with cholinesterase inhibitor treatment, and prolongation of end stage improved behavioural function with memantine.

In most dementias the patients themselves will not necessarily be aware of benefit but the majority of carers will notice an uplift in mental facility, that will show itself in a variety of ways. Comments such as: 'He's more like his old self', or 'He takes an interest in the newspaper properly again instead of just scanning it' and 'She joins in at bowls again now and enjoys it' are typically reported by carers of treated patients when asked about the effects of drugs. This benefit in concentration, mental ability and confidence at mental and physical tasks may not show itself until mid-range or upper-range dose is achieved, but will be evident within 5 days of dose change. Prolonged trials of 4–8 weeks at each dose are justified to allow a carer to observe performance in a wide range of situations, which they will readily report, for example:

'He actually paid attention when our daughter came with her little boy at half term.' The unifying principle of all neurotransmitter replacement treatments is 'stoking the furnace', by which we mean continue titrating treatment until a threshold is crossed where benefit is obtained. Once benefit occurs drugs should be further titrated to obtain higher benefit and all drugs should be used to the maximum tolerated dose. There is no point titrating above recommended dose levels, as more than 90% of available acetyl or butyryl cholinesterase enzyme sites are occupied by the drugs at maximum therapeutic levels. This means only side effects accrue beyond this point, without further benefit.

Some GPs may have come across the idea that the hallucinatory symptoms of dementia with Lewy bodies will particularly respond to treatment. However in the authors' experience this has not been borne out in practice and the positive effects are unpredictable. In rapid eye movement (REM) sleep disorder associated with dementia with Lewy bodies, the effect of drug treatment is varied. However, the authors have occasionally seen a complete resolution of this agitated dreaming state on cholinesterase inhibitor treatment. More rarely a paradoxical dose-related precipitation of REM sleep disturbance can occur in Alzheimer's disease patients when treated with these drugs. Impaired levels of daytime arousal are a feature of dementia with Lewy bodies and can sometimes can be improved by cholinesterase inhibitors but there does not seem to be a corresponding similar benefit in Alzheimer's disease on daytime naps and apathy.

The fronto-temporal lobe dementia case history in Chapter 1 illustrates how a brief upward swing in confidence, mood and function can be achieved with treatment. Typically however, this is subsequently and rapidly swamped by the developing behavioural abnormality, impaired speech and swallowing as well as peripheral neurological signs.

The role of the Mini Mental State Examination (MMSE)

Nowadays serial testing is most often done using the Mini Mental State Examination although it was not designed or validated for successive testing originally. It may have a one to two point variability, known as the test–retest reliability, by the same interviewer. There is also often considerably more disparity between interviewers of as much as 4 points, so called inter-rater reliability. The causes of this variability are very similar to the wide variation in blood pressure measurements for the same patient in different settings.

In the Mini Mental State Examination interviewer technique needs to be applied accurately and consistently. The interview setting should avoid allowing patients to appeal to a relative using eye contact or direct questioning which can distort results. The tester also needs to take care not to use incorrect explicit or generalised interventions. Many clinicians will intuitively use non-verbal prompts such as making encouraging noises, nodding, or saying '*well done*' for correct answers, out of a desire to facilitate the patient and make them feel more at ease. Of course this alters a patient's confidence doing the test, and the reduced anxiety often improves score. The converse is also true and a strictly applied test condition with silence and no prompting or choices, will at times freeze a patient or cause them to become irritable or even break down in tears. When a test has to be aborted to spare the patient's feelings or those of a relative, the time and suffering already imposed is wasted and a negative cycle has been set up between the patient, carer and GP. The best approach is to try to ensure that the same person does the testing each time with the patient in as near an identical style and setting, alone in the room without relatives. If this is done then the variations in personal style matter less as what one is looking for at 3- or 6-month intervals is evidence of change. This may be on a spectrum of upward improvement of between plus 2 to plus 6 points and maintenance of score over baseline, for 9 months to 2 years. At the other end of the response spectrum a GP may see unimpeded deterioration at a relatively fast rate such as, minus 1–2 points every 3–6 months, despite treatment. In pharmaceutical trials and local clinician-based clinical audit the majority of patients show stability or improvement, but with average modest score changes of plus 1 to 3 points. These benefits are maintained for 6–18 months and then the scores deteriorate by 2–4 points per year to near baseline eventually.

How to decide when to stop treatment

Withdrawing treatments from patients can have psychological implications for the whole family. Therefore it is worth taking some time to explain both the rationale and the process. As with so many aspects of dementia management, engaging the carers in the drug management will make them feel informed and better able to cope. It will also mean they can reliably report changes to their GP and other healthcare professionals to the benefit of the patient. Furthermore, carers who are well prepared and know they will be reviewing the situation with the doctor, will be calmer overall and less likely to make emergency calls to the surgery.

From a practical point of view, GPs can factor in attempting drug withdrawal either upon request or at a suitable agreed point in treatment. This might be after 3 or 4 years, or when the patient undergoes sudden significant deterioration, such as with a TIA, infection or fall, after which they fail to recover most of their function. Other circumstances might include the transfer to residential care, or when the obvious terminal stage of illness has begun some 3 months or more before death. Withdrawal can be rapid, over 48 hours, and should be maintained for 5–10 days before deciding whether to restart the drug or not.

As in Mr Ashley's case, if the patient were still benefiting from their treatment they will show obvious cognitive or behavioural deterioration within a day or two of withdrawal, and the drug can be immediately reinstated. A more subtle effect can be monitored over 10–14 days, during which time carers should be asked to keep simple diaries to record isolated behaviours such as agitation, weeping, pinching or punching. This allows the carers to gauge whether there is a more subtle general downward shift in the patient's condition including their level of attention, apathy, eye contact and overall happiness, when the drug is stopped. If so, again the treatment can be reinstated. For the best demonstration of benefit or adverse effect, an 'a-b-a' model of patient trial can be undertaken. This means: stop treatment, monitor, restart treatment for 2 weeks, monitor, then stop again for 2 weeks. This will give powerful information even about rare benefits and adverse effects and a decision can then be made in joint discussion with carers, family and others involved. This is an opportune moment to discuss the expected problems in the next phase of illness.

When to stop has been a subject of debate since treatment began. The early 1997 protocols of the Maudsley Hospital, UK, suggested a 3-month trial and if no benefit was seen the drug should be stopped. This proved unpopular, over-constricting and unworkable. In contrast in a few sympathetic NHS trusts and in private practice it was possible to undertake prolonged treatment. The clinical evidence on long-term treatment accrued faster than trial evidence, particularly in the US. This is because no pharmaceutical company or public body worldwide would fund long-term trials given the problems of obtaining and maintaining patient numbers and excluding other serious illness. There was also the issue of persuading patients and carers to continue to accept placebo treatment against the backdrop public furore about non-availability of treatment generally. It was the drive for assessment of cost effectiveness by public health funders that led to trials in the UK, which did not factor in the commercial risk to a drug from unexpected long-term findings. The NHS-funded 'AD 2000' trial in the UK from 2000 to 2003 showed continued benefit of those taking donepezil over placebo even after 3 years. More recently another independent UK group at King's College London, showed benefit over 10 years.

What guidance can GPs give about side effects?

Emma Price was a 74-year-old widow who was prone to weeping depression and feelings of uselessness after the death of her active husband. This was worse since her only daughter had emigrated to France with her family. After 10 years of intermittent treatment for anxiety and depression with an SSRI and anxiety management, her GP, Dr Ditchling, found her memory was deteriorating and therefore requested review by an Old Age Psychiatrist. Mrs Price was diagnosed with early Alzheimer's disease and was given an introductory dose of the acetyl cholinesterase inhibitor, galantamine 4 mg once daily for 2 weeks, which was achieved by cutting an 8 mg tablet in half. When this was increased to twice daily Mrs Price experienced a host of side effects, including hypothermia, diarrhoea, nausea and vomiting, muscle cramps, sialorrhoea, rhinorrhoea, lacrimation, agitation and nocturnal confusion. This remarkable range and depth of cholinergic side effects is almost unheard of at such low doses of the drug. For understandable reasons, Mrs Price asked to be taken off galantamine and was managed in the community without drug therapy.

The above experience illustrates a research finding described by the teams such as Terry and deKosky respectively, where the proliferation of cholinergic synaptic sites and increased cholinergic generative enzyme (choline acetyltransferase) is thought to sometimes occur in early Alzheimer's disease or in the possibly related condition of mild cognitive impairment. This may explain this sensitivity to side effects as there may be more of the cholinergic system for the drug to act on.

The data sheets issued with drug treatments are invaluable for the patient and their family in terms of knowing what is possible, but all too often they have difficulty differentiating common side effects from very rare ones. For this reason it is important to talk about possible side effects with patients and their nearest carer as they may forget. It is also worth writing the information down for them so that they can refer back to the advice at a later date when they are alone and possibly frightened.

Non-drug therapies in dementia

A range of non-drug therapies are used in patients with dementia. As with many complementary therapies, opinions vary as to their effectiveness but it can be argued that any intervention which improves a patient's mood or quality of life is worth using. Families also often feel better when these therapies are used, as they provide a nurturing, often sensory, environment for the patient.

Box 3.1 Side effects of cholinergic drugs

Common side effects:
- centrally mediated nausea, vomiting and diarrhoea.
  Rarer side effects:
- small muscle cramps, sweating, over-sedation, headaches and hypothermia;
- vulnerable patients may develop bradycardia and syncope.
  Rarer but serious side effects:
- prolonged bleeding from an active peptic ulcer although less likely today due to rapid prescribing of anti-ulcer drugs;
- prolongation of cardiac conduction with sino-atrial or atrio-ventricular block and subsequent dysrhythmia.

Cognitive stimulation therapy. This uses multi-source cognitive stimulation, in a social setting, to attempt to activate latent cognitive abilities. There is some research evidence that it improves mood or behaviour but not necessarily cognition. However there is little evidence as to how long its effect lasts.

Aromatherapy. This may have a beneficial effect and there is one good randomised controlled study, using lemon balm (*Melissa officinalis*) for 4 weeks, which showed an effect on agitation.

Music therapy or other multi-sensory stimulation can produce a pleasurable effect and improve mood while it is ongoing, but the long-term effect remains unproven.

Physical exercise. Although there is no good research evidence so far, it clearly helps patients in a social context and also those who have always been active.

Reminiscence therapy. This also often improves patients' mood and also works well in a group setting.

Validation therapy. This means validating a patient's subjective experience. For example, if a therapist tells a demented patient who asks tearfully for her mother that her parent is long dead, that is reality orientation therapy (ROT). However if they say, '*I see you miss her very much*', that is validation therapy. Validation therapy is considered kinder than reality orientation therapy but there is no evidence that it is more effective in improving mood, behaviour or cognition in the long term. In the example given, the patient may know that the parent they love is dead, but their memory impairment aids their reluctance to admit it.

Key points

- Drug treatment for dementia varies across the country, but in principle should be offered to all patients.
- Donepezil is the most commonly prescribed anticholinergic drug seen in general practice.
- Memantine has a relatively safe cardiac side effect profile making it a useful drug in at-risk patients with dementia.
- Rivastigmine is licensed for Parkinson's disease dementia.
- The Mini Mental State Examination, conducted correctly, is a useful test to establish a baseline and monitor the effects of treatment.
- Carers commonly report a significant uplift in mental ability when patients are actively treated.
- Warning patients and carers about potential side effects in writing is advisable before initiating dementia treatments.
- Asking carers to keep a diary will help doctors to detect relapses during drug withdrawal.
- Complementary therapies can have a beneficial effect on patients and their families.

Reference

Clarke, N.A. & Francis, P.T. (2005) Cholinergic and glutamatergic drugs in Alzheimer's disease therapy. *Expert Review of Neurotherapeutics*, **5**(5), 671–682.

Francis, P.T., Parsons, C.G. and Jones, R.W. (2012). Rationale for combining glutamatergic and cholinergic approaches in the symptomatic treatment of Alzheimer's disease. [online] http://www.medscape.com/viewpublication/21461. *Expert Review of Neurotherapeutics*, **12**(11), 1351–1365.

Chapter 4 **Emergency management of dementia**

While it is true that emergency situations in dementia may be unavoidable, it is also true that the more educated and supported patients and their relatives are, the more likely they will be to cope with sudden dramas. This means that once the diagnosis of dementia has been confirmed, usually with the help of a specialist, educating patients and carers about the likely course of the disease will prepare them for the emergence of new sets of symptoms as they arise. This in turn will mean they are less panicked by acute events.

Contingency planning is also best undertaken in advance of the condition progressing. This will include an understanding of what medication, or types of medication, may be required from time to time and what care services will be available when they are needed. Discussions about when to move the patient to more manageable accommodation or how to provide increased support at home are all best undertaken early rather than late in the disease. If they are not needed then that is a bonus, but it's worth remembering that patients and relatives are on 'catch up' compared to their GP and may never have thought about some of the situations they will now face. They may also be unprepared for the fluidity and pace of change which comes with dementia. A couple who have lived together for 60 years may have precisely planned what to do should one of them die, but will not have considered how they will cope should one of them end up living in a care home. Allowing patients sufficient time to digest, not only the implications of the diagnosis, but also the options to deal with the inevitable changes in lifestyle, will make the GP's management much easier. Effectively the GP and dementia specialists are expecting patients and their families to 'manage change' as it arises. Most of the population find this difficult at the best of times, and it is a very tall order

How to Manage Dementia in General Practice, First Edition. Nicholas Clarke, Farine Clarke, and Denzil Edwards.
© 2013 John Wiley & Sons Ltd. Published 2013 by John Wiley & Sons, Ltd.

in this age group. This is probably the main reason why dementia care can appear to be disproportionately stressful in capable families, many of whom GPs have managed without difficulty for several years.

In addition to the GP and specialist in Old Age Psychiatry, dementia experts such as Admiral Nurses and other members of the multidisciplinary team, who are discussed in detail in Chapter 6, will all help to prepare patients and carers for emergencies as they arise.

For the purpose of this book, all references are to the Mental Capacity Act (2005) and the Mental Health Act (1983 as amended in 2007).

What constitutes an emergency presentation of dementia?

Mrs Ringmer was an 83-year-old widow who lived with her rather aloof middle-aged son. Despite her age, Mrs Ringmer had minimal dealings with her GP, Dr Smith, and a good relationship with her neighbours who considered her to be a reliable and conscientious person. However one evening, Mrs Ringmer appeared at the local convenience store in her underwear and proceeded to argue with the shoppers.

The police were called and, after a brief assessment, decided she was not a danger to herself or to others and took her home. They also informed social services, who in turn passed her details to the Mental Health Services for Older People team the next day. However, before they visited, Mrs. Ringmer left her home in her nightdress again. This time her neighbour picked her up and called her GP surgery.

Dr Smith found Mrs Ringmer to be confused and suffering with marked auditory hallucinations. He was unable to obtain a collateral history as her son was absent. Examination revealed no obvious cause for her confusion and, after sending routine blood and urine samples to the laboratory, he referred her to the physicians for possible admission.

The admitting team diagnosed acute on chronic confusion but could not find a cause and discharged Mrs Ringmer the following day with back-up from social services.

After a few weeks social services contacted Dr Smith to say that Mrs Ringmer was continuing to act inappropriately. She had dialled 999 to complain about non-existent intruders and asked the dustmen into the house because she was 'worried about the children'.

This time Dr Smith contacted the consultant Old Age Psychiatrist, who visited Mrs Ringmer at home. He found that Mrs Ringmer was intermittently confused: at times she was aware of her address, at others she thought she was in Somerset where she had lived 30 years ago. Although she was not hallucinat-

*ing at the time, she had good insight and did recall experiencing visual hallu-
cinations. She agreed to admission to hospital for investigation and observation
where the eventual diagnosis of dementia with Lewy bodies was made.*

The above case illustrates many of the features of an 'emergency' presentation of dementia. GPs are rarely called to a dementia emergency where the
patient is violent for the first time or throwing the television out of the
window. Mrs Ringmer is a more common example of a so-called acute
presentation of the condition. It is not unusual for a concerned neighbour
to call a doctor to an elderly patient's home for the first time because they
are behaving oddly.

The onset of dementia in itself is not acute but appears to be so because
patients who live alone or have no family carers are not brought to their GP's
attention as their symptoms develop. This means only when a drama occurs
and the police are involved do investigations into the condition begin.

Referral to the physicians in the first instance is also more common, as in
this case, because the patient's symptoms may well mimic that of an acute
confusional state, which is far more common in the elderly. In turn the
physicians will typically refer the patient back into the community or request
the Old Age Psychiatrist to carry out an in-patient assessment prior to discharge. Understandably, GPs may find the process frustrating, particularly if
no one takes ownership of the problem and the mental health team fails to
attend quickly.

In some patients who appear to present with acute symptoms, careful
questioning will reveal a history of memory or other cognitive impairment
which had not been brought to the GP's attention. As has been already said,
this may be because they live alone, or because the patient or relatives
thought the symptoms were very mild or a natural part of ageing. Fear or
denial by the family as well as the patient will all contribute to delayed
presentation.

Acute confusional state

The authors acknowledge that GPs are well versed in the management of
acute confusional state in the elderly and will readily make diagnosis *in situ*,
using simple diagnostic tools such as a stethoscope and urinary dip-sticks.
This section will therefore deal with true presentations of dementia.

Patients with dementing illness are more susceptible to acute confusion
from any given stimulus. However, the overriding rule when managing
someone with pre-existing dementia, is to treat the acute state as one would
any other elderly patient. By this we mean do not allow management to be
diverted by the fact there is pre-existing dementia. This also means that if a

GP feels there is a treatable physical cause for the emergency presentation which cannot be managed at home, then hospital admission via A & E, or through the admitting Old Age Physicians is indicated.

There are an increasing number of GPs with a great deal of experience of the elderly, who are able to divert their confused patient to the mental health services in the first instance, rather than the second. This means their patients avoid the extensive tests which tend to occur at presentation of acute confusion. Clearly this has time and cost savings as well as a degree of clinical satisfaction for the referring GP who has by bypassed negative tests. In the authors' experience GPs with this level of experience are only able to refer a new case in this way once every 4–5 years on average.

Box 4.1 Common causes of acute confusion in the elderly

- Infection, for example respiratory or urinary tract
- Cardiovascular disease, for example angina, heart failure
- Cerebrovascular event
- Anaemia
- New onset or exacerbated diabetes
- Other endocrine disease, for example hypothyroidism
- Worsening of COPD
- Constipation
- Drug intoxication

Box 4.2 Rarer causes of acute confusion in elderly

- Complex drug effect: the sedative and confusing effects of anxiolytic and hypnotic drugs. Benzodiazepines cause confusion by themselves, which will be made worse in forgetful patients who take excessive doses
- Acute stroke without neurological signs
- An uncomplicated painless bony injury however minor, typically a pubic ramus or rib
- Pain such as from chronic osteoarthritis or shingles
- Metabolic disturbances such as hyponatraemia, sometimes secondary to antidepressants
- Lengthy travel by car or air, such as driving to Scotland from Kent or flying to an unaccustomed adverse climate such as Australia or a boat to Bergen
- Major changes in emotional environment such as the death of an old friend
- Grief for a dead pet
- Major changes in domiciliary environment, including staying with relatives or moving rooms within a care home

A practical approach to the acute presentation

Do I need to be there immediately or can I visit later in the day?

There is no corresponding situation to a heart attack emergency in dementia, but to help GPs triage in their own minds how quickly they need to respond it is worth assessing three questions: How vulnerable is the person calling? How much can the GP help if they go immediately? If the GP can't help who could attend instead? In the latter situation the GP might feel it appropriate to ask the community psychiatric nurse (CPN) first to assess the situation, particularly if they have more time. Thus, if the patient is known to the local mental health services team then the GP might request they visit first.

Although GPs are often willing to be the first to visit a patient in an emergency there are actually circumstances where it may not be appropriate. If the patient is uncontrollably violent, or they have run away and their whereabouts are unknown then clearly the GP cannot attend. Also in some situations it may be unsafe for the GP to use their usual clinical armoury, for example if the patient is at the side of the road then administering drugs becomes dangerous. Finally if the GP simply does not have time for a lengthy visit, perhaps because afternoon surgery is about to start, but the patient still requires urgent attention, then they should also consider calling in other help.

What precautions should I take with the patient?

It is vital that GPs take appropriate precautions to protect themselves when seeing a patient with dementia in an emergency for the first time. Although sustained, directed violence towards doctors is extremely rare in this group it is still worth being safe. Patients with dementing illness can show similar degrees of excitement as those with acute schizophrenia, mania or mixed affective disorder, especially in acute confusional states. Those who are suffering from early-onset dementia are generally physically stronger and pose a greater risk than the elderly. Having said that, just because a patient is elderly and appears to be frail or has been living with a very frail spouse without harming them, does not preclude them from inflicting damage on a stranger.

Outside confusional states, patients suffering from persecutory delusions are a particular risk, although health professionals are less likely to be part of the patient's delusional system.

GPs should employ the usual precautions they would in the surgery, like ensuring the exit is not blocked by the patient, waiting for assistance before conducting an examination and removing potential weapons including walking sticks.

In rare cases relatives can also pose a physical threat and this should not be underestimated where younger relatives are stressed and have a history of violence. For many elderly people their dog is their closest companion and can respond aggressively to anyone appearing to 'attack' their master during the examination. In turn a confused owner may cry out when handled or be unable to control their pet as they would normally. Therefore dogs, however docile, should be removed. The overall aim in the examination, as well as establishing a diagnosis is to ensure the patient does not become more agitated or excited.

Who do I call (day and night)?

It is perfectly legitimate for any GP who is at all concerned about safety to call the emergency services, including the police, at the same time as setting off to visit a patient at home. In working hours they can also contact the duty worker on the local mental health services for older people team or the Old Age Psychiatrist directly. Speaking with the consultant on the phone will help to decide on the best course of action. GPs may request a joint visit to the patient with a CPN or psychiatrist, not least because team members typically welcome the chance to access the GP's knowledge of the patient first hand. It is far better for them to have a calm introduction to the patient via the GP in a stressed situation. Currently, a good time for joint home assessments is between 12 and 2.30 pm when GPs have scheduled visits and team members are unlikely to be in meetings or ward reviews.

At night or at weekends the local mental health crisis intervention team receptionist, duty CPN or equivalent should be able to triage the case for immediate further assessment.

Sectioning under the Mental Health Act

It is rare for patients with dementia to require assessment under the Mental Health Act, but if it is thought necessary then the local mental health crisis team should liaise between the GP, the on-call senior mental health social worker or nurse, the approved mental health practitioner (AMHP) who is responsible for completing the section and transferring the patient to a local hospital, and the duty consultant psychiatrist. Sometimes an independent Mental Health Act Section 12 approved doctor is used if the patient's own GP is unavailable for the assessment. The AMHP will arrange this from a list of doctors kept by the relevant regional NHS licensing authority. The GP or their substitute Section 12 doctor will attend either with the other medical consultant or with the AMHP. The medical recommendations may be completed separately as long as they are within 5 days of each other. According to the Act one of the doctors should have prior knowledge of the patient, but this is honoured more in the breach than in the observance.

Section 13 of the Mental Health Act 1983 still stands and Local Social Service Authorities are obliged to arrange for an AMHP to consider the case of any patient within their area if asked to do so by or on behalf of the nearest relative. In practice, this does not mean that the local authority can ignore anyone else! The same Section lays down that social services must arrange for an AMHP to consider the case of any patient within their area if they have reason to believe that an application for detention in hospital may need to be made in respect of the patient. Obviously, a call from a GP or psychiatrist about the patient's condition is going to give them plenty of 'reason to believe'.

Having said that, there is nothing in law to stop social services from delegating this task, and many have done so. This makes some sense now that AMHPs are not just social workers, like the former approved social workers, but can be nurses, psychologists and so on. The AMHP on duty is likely to be within the local mental health crisis team and that is the team which must be contacted. Obviously, social services would be remiss if they did not ensure callers speak with the right team promptly when contacted by someone who is unaware of the new arrangements.

This all means that GPs who cannot get hold of an AMHP, can request a section assessment directly from social services and the onus is on them to contact the right party for the area.

If the GP, as the patient's advocate, initiates the sectioning process, they are often unable to guarantee that they will still be on duty when the section is finalised. This may raise concern that the patient will experience nighttime delays in an A & E assessment unit, or be inappropriately placed in a psychiatric emergency unit dominated by restless and frightened younger adults. In these circumstances a discussion earlier in the day with the relevant consultant Old Age Psychiatrist will help to ensure the patient is seen sooner and their eventual placement is more appropriate.

Section 2 of the Mental Health Act allows for a period of medical and nursing assessment including that of the effect of treatment for up to 28 days. Section 3 assumes that the diagnosis is known and is a treatment order for up to 6 months and which can be used where the patient is well known to the treating team and the course of action reasonably clear.

A conflict of interest may arise between NHS organisations and social services. Once a patient is detained on Section 3 they are entitled on discharge to what is known as section 117 (Mental Health Act) aftercare provided by the local authority regardless of the patient's own means. Conversely if the patient is not detained on Section 3 if they have means, they do not qualify for this provision and will have to pay for themselves or seek entitlement to NHS continuing care. A family may be reluctant to commit their relative for up to 6 months, but this should not be an obstacle. A skilled AMHP or knowledgeable GP can explain how Section 3 offers the same protections as Section 2, and is unlikely to extend in use much beyond an initial settling period of a few days or weeks.

What do I look for if I suspect an undiagnosed dementia?

Miss Elizabeth Baxter was a 90-year-old lady with history of arthritis of both knees which impaired her mobility and stability, together with long-standing hypertension. She moved into a care home and was taken on to Dr Gin's list although she suffered a fall before his first visit. Dr Gin attended immediately and the staff told him that Mrs Baxter appeared to lose consciousness briefly before falling. On examination no neurological signs were found, nor any external sign of head injury and Dr Gin sent Mrs Baxter to A & E. To his surprise, no neuroimaging was undertaken and she was sent back to the home. On her return she was anxious and uncharacteristically bad tempered. She had visual hallucinations and muddled thinking, misidentifying objects like a wicker chair as a commode. Dr Gin took a midstream specimen of urine (MSU) and started antibiotics, on the assumption of a UTI, before referring Mrs Baxter to the mental health services for older people (MHSOP) team. Aside from her hypertensive history he also informed the team that a CT brain scan done 3 years earlier had shown subcortical small vessel changes.

Although there were no relatives at this stage, the Old Age Psychiatrist eventually spoke with Mrs Baxter's nephew who said his aunt had been suffering from mild memory impairment for about a year.

On cognitive examination, Miss Baxter was found to have a patchy and variable memory impairment, in full consciousness. She knew where she was, but was unable to name the residential home. The psychiatrist diagnosed small-vessel or mixed vascular dementia, and recommended a trial of treatment with an atypical neuroleptic with appropriate caution about the risk of side effects.

The above case demonstrates that it is easier for the GP who knows a patient's background condition to distinguish what is new in an emergency situation. However, unlike in physical illness, when encountering a dementia patient for the first time, the signs of the illness are often in the surroundings rather than directly on the patient. Observational clues appear on first sight of a property if the patient lives alone. Typically the front garden is overgrown, the paint peeling and fences are damaged. Internal chaos may take the form of 'organised clutter' with neat piles of paperwork waiting to be dealt with by a once capable and conscientious person whose overall abilities may fluctuate, but fall short of dealing effectively with administration. The interior may smell of animals and faeces. Signs of neglect may extend to the patient, who can be unkempt and may also show signs of starvation and untreated minor injuries or ulcers.

In emergency situations the carer may not have had time to mask every aspect of the patient's illness, so although they may appear tidy and the accommodation clean, GPs may still feel something isn't quite right, this may be as subtle as the odour of stale milk in tea or a full dustbin bag that has not been put outside the house.

Unlike many elderly patients, piles of unused medication will not be stockpiled in the bathroom cabinet, because these patients have not been in contact with their GP.

None of these signs are infallible in terms of diagnosis, nor do they always occur, and they can be present with other conditions, but evidence of neglect is often a feature of dementia, particularly in those living alone.

In the absence of family, neighbours are useful as they notice changes in behaviour and signs of memory impairment and often have contact details for the relatives. In these circumstances a telephone conversation with the family may reveal simple changes, like the grandmother who never forgets a grandchild's birthday suddenly sending two cards on the wrong dates or writing the wrong names. They are also likely to report previous instances of mistaken identity, such as widower mistaking his daughter for his late wife. Relatives may have viewed all of these minor problems as insignificant, but they now become invaluable to the diagnosis.

GPs can take time during this first emergency visit to extend the positives in the history while automatically excluding the negatives via urine dipsticks and respiratory examination for cardiac failure. At this stage of proceedings, it doesn't really matter if the patient has a few apparently toxic symptoms such as visual hallucinations or a gross disorientation in time and place, akin to delirium. This is because as long as there is a clean history, the way the patient progresses through the next phase is not pre-determined and does not appear to be directly proportional to any particular intervention. This means that however odd the picture, GPs have time to reach their conclusions and doing so may result in a better outcome if they correctly divert that patient to the mental health team rather than into casualty.

How likely is this to progress to the patient having to leave the home situation?

GPs who are in doubt about whether a patient should remain at home can talk with the Old Age Psychiatrist who might also discuss which follow-up services are available in the area to visit in the immediate term. If the patient does remain at home then they need to be in a stable, manageable state and their carer, who may themselves be elderly, needs to be confident they can manage. If the carer and family can cope then it is worth ensuring the mental health service for older people team is also involved and can check on the patient immediately post 'emergency' and also monitor progress with the GP to ensure the situation remains stable.

All support services including the CPNs and Admiral Nurses can visit the family regularly after the event to continue monitoring the patient and also oversee any medication.

In situations where the carer cannot cope, or when the GP has tried to manage the situation but it blows up repeatedly, admission to hospital or a care facility may be the only option.

What drugs are safe to use?

If the demented patient is so distressed, agitated or violent to make adequate physical examination impossible, acute sedation may be required. It also may be needed in sequel if the patient needs acute treatment, or admission to hospital.

The order of use of drugs is as follows.

Lorazepam is the short-acting sedative drug of choice. In elderly patients with dementia it is usually required at only a low dose, such as 0.5–1.0 mg. The overall safety profile is generally good, but respiratory depression, especially in those at risk, and in higher doses, is a dangerous side effect. Typically a 0.5 mg dose can be taken orally and, if ineffective within 20 minutes, repeated at 0.5 mg or 1 mg and so on to a total dose of 2 mg within the hour. No further dosage should be given for 6–8 hours. To enhance the speed of action, and avoid inadvertent under-dosing by medication spillage or loss by the patient, intramuscular lorazepam in a similar dose range can be used instead.

If lorazepam is insufficiently calming then neuroleptics can be used in conjunction with the short-acting benzodiazepine, albeit with varying degrees of success and adverse effects. Sometimes a 24–48-hour trial period of lorazepam 0.5–2 mg PRN TDS (up to 8-hourly) causes over-sedation, but a lower dose is ineffective. In those circumstances the introduction of a concurrent neuroleptic allows GPs to reduce the benzodiazepine to a non-sedating level.

The principles governing antipsychotic use include employing them in low doses if at all, and allowing them sufficient time to take effect, which is typically a week or 10 days, before increasing the dose. They should be reviewed frequently, and used for as short a time as possible. Attempts to discontinue them should be made within 2 months. Antipsychotic medication is strongly contraindicated in dementia with Lewy bodies because of the risk of extrapyramidal side effects which can be life threatening. This means that antipsychotics in dementia with Lewy bodies should be used with extreme caution and this is best attempted only in secondary care.

For oral administration and more gently graded effect, oral low-dose atypical antipsychotic drugs are therefore the next consideration (Table 4.1).

Amisulpiride (Solian, Sanofi Aventis) is derived from one of the least potent and least side effect beset of the older typical antipsychotics, sulpiride. It probably retains some of the antidepressant or activating effect of the drug that were in the past observed to improve negative symptoms of schizophrenia in younger patients at very much higher doses, which was up to 1200 mg of sulpiride per day. Like quetiapine, amisulpiride is not available as a parenteral preparation. However in an emergency it has the potential for GP use in very low doses by dividing tablets into half or quarter. Some patients settle on amisulpiride 25 mg, which is half of the smallest 50 mg tablet, or quetiapine (Seroquel, AstraZeneca) 12.5 mg, which is half of the smallest 25 mg tablet, and even amisulpiride approximately 12.5 mg, which is a quarter tablet. Typical initial regimes are amisulpiride 25 mg BD increasing to 50 mg BD after 2 days if ineffective, or quetiapine 12.5 mg BD increasing to 25 mg BD. Liquid preparations can be substituted for amisulpiride but not quetiapine, once the situation permits. However a liquid drug is not usually a self-administration option for a cognitively impaired patient living alone or with some lay carers. Quetiapine has received some adverse notices, on account of its potential to produce abnormalities of heart conduction, such as QTc prolongation, but this rarely progresses to the dangerous arrhythmia of torsade de pointes. In contrast to the clinical experience of Old Age Psychiatrists and specialist in-patient units, the few and small-scale controlled trials of these drugs for behavioural and psychological symptoms of dementia, tend to provide little further evidence to support their use in agitation and psychosis.

The remaining two commonly considered atypical antipsychotics, risperidone (Risperdal, Jannsen) and olanzapine (Zyprexa, Lilly), must both be viewed in the cautious light of their makers' post-marketing surveillance findings and subsequent Cochrane review warnings. Both have been shown to be associated with increased, albeit low, incidence of cerebrovascular events in patients with dementia. The reasons for this are unknown. This effect is not known to extend to their use in the non-demented elderly, but caution is advised with any older person with concurrent vascular risk factors or a previous history of stroke.

Risperidone is the only antipsychotic licensed for the treatment of behavioural and psychological symptoms of dementia (BPSD) in dementia, and again should be tried at well below normal adult dose. We suggest an initial

Table 4.1 Available presentations of some atypical antipsychotics compared to haliperidol.

	Amisulpride	Aripiprazole	Olanzapine	Quetiapine	Risperidone	Haloperidol
Tablet	✓	✓	✓	✓	✓	✓
M/R tablet				✓		
Orodispersible tablet		✓	✓		✓	
Liquid (syrup or solution)	✓	✓			✓	✓
IM injection		✓	✓		✓	✓
Depot injection			✓			✓

dose of 0.25 mg (250 micrograms) risperidone OD or BD increasing to risperidone 1 mg OD to BD. On a further note of caution, the authors have observed the widely considered drawback with this drug of increased extrapyramidal adverse effects. Risperdal Consta is a unique extended-release depot version atypical antipsychotic which is rarely used in dementia because of concern over side effects vulnerability. However this intramuscular treatment may be useful for GPs with a patient who settles well and cannot manage without this or another antipsychotic drug but in whom behaviour or geography make compliance a problem. Research supports its use in aggression in patients with dementia.

Olanzapine is a powerful antipsychotic drug and also a suitable ingestible alternative. Dosage starts at 2.5 mg PRN OD and is increased in 2.5 mg increments every 2 days up to 10 mg per day. Whilst less likely to cause extrapyramidal effects than risperidone in the authors' opinion, it is worth being aware of its anticognitive anticholinergic effects, not least because these are not an issue in others members of this group of drugs. Doctors should consider olanzapine's metabolic effects and discuss these with the patient and family if they anticipate using it for more than 8–12 weeks. Although weight gain and impaired glycaemic control may not unduly concern a patient with BPSD, given what we know about the interrelationship between cardiac compartment vascular risk factors and Alzheimer degeneration, they are best avoided.

Haloperidol, the short-acting butyrophenone antipsychotic, remains the drug of choice for immediate symptom resolution by oral or parenteral means. It is one of the older typical antipsychotic drugs with relatively safe and predictable effects. The drug's use in the acute situation is countenanced by NICE, but, like all antipsychotics, should be used only for severe distress or where there is a risk of physical harm. Oral treatment at dose of 0.5 mg (500 micrograms) should be offered in the first instance, repeated after half an hour if ineffective. A typical daily dose is 0.5–3 mg orally for an elderly patient.

Intramuscular treatment should be started with a single dose of haloperidol 2 mg, up to a maximum of 5 mg in exceptional circumstances. If ineffective alone or in conjunction with low-dose benzodiazepine, the antipsychotic dose can be repeated after 1 hour. It should then be continued up to three times a day at the lower end of this dose range. For example haloperidol 2 mg BD-TDS for 3 days initially with a PRN option of haloperidol 5 mg single dose supplement IM where needed.

The prescribing doctor should ensure that the total administered daily dose of haloperidol does not exceed 15 mg. In patients who are previously drug naïve to an antipsychotic and have existing organic brain disease the dose of haloperidol 10 mg should probably not be exceeded for more than

3–5 days without specialist review and supervision. This is because of the increased likelihood of serious adverse effects.

Generally with antipsychotic treatments extrapyramidal side effects, although quite common, are very rarely life threatening, while the serious cardiovascular side effects are rare. Mild induction of liver enzymes is sufficiently common to be unremarkable especially with the older typical drugs, and it is unusual to find clinical evidence of hepatic symptoms. It is worth warning carers to look out for neurological signs such as paradoxical akathisia or inner restlessness where the patient seems to be made more aimlessly motile after each dose of antipsychotic. Treatment discontinuation nearly always confirms the diagnosis. Delayed evolution of limb, trunk or facial movement abnormalities, a writhing twisting movement of the limbs or rapid repeated lip pursing, can be a serious and sometimes irreversible effect of prolonged neuroleptic treatment, requiring specialist advice on drug changes. However the GP, when discussing the potential for tardive dyskinesias with the family and patient before treatment, is likely to find that they take a pragmatic view of the risks. Even if irreversible, the abnormal movements pale beside the distress and danger of an agitated psyche in a dementia patient.

With antipsychotics and even antidepressants the risk of a very rare but potentially lethal neuroleptic malignant syndrome may be more likely in the already compromised brain. This is more likely to present as body temperature and muscle tone dysregulation with autonomic instability, rather than mildly altered conscious levels before the onset of stupor or coma. Grossly elevated creatine kinase (CK) levels help to point to the diagnosis. Treatment is immediate neuroleptic discontinuation, and urgent medical support for the somatic symptoms.

The authors have not observed acute painful torticollis in dementia patients on antipsychotic drugs, in contrast to its sporadic occurrence in younger psychotic inpatients. This may be because the latter are on fast-escalation, higher-dose drug regimes. Should a GP come across this in a dementia patient after initiating a course of neuroleptic therapy, the management is the same, namely antipsychotic dose reduction and single dose administration of procyclidine 5 mg IM or orally.

When to not medicate?
Drugs are one of the key tools GPs bring to a distressed situation involving a family and patient with dementia. However there are many factors which can cause agitation in these patients, including carer abuse. Therefore the family expectation that drugs will be used should not be satisfied without further consideration. Rare abuse takes the form of physical violence, which is often surreptitious and signs include fingertip bruising and unexplained

injuries. More common abuse relates to the 'sins of omission' of care, which can be accidental or otherwise. Examples include a failure to give medication or to feed a patient or ensure they are sufficiently warm.

Repeated critical questioning and inappropriate feedback from carers is punitive in cases of dementia and results in understandable frustration and agitation in the patient. GPs will witness carers playing this out in front of them with angry comments like, '*you've asked me that ten times*', in response to a patient's question. This makes GPs among the best professionals to detect this form of abuse which is by no means mild.

When to review the patient post-emergency

When a GP leaves the emergency situation it is useful to give a contact number for the carers to call should the patient fail to settle over the next 4–5 hours. This allows the GP to leave while at the same time reassuring the family that they have not been abandoned.

If the GP hears nothing immediately, it is worth reviewing the patient in the next 2–3 days, by which time any oversedation or extrapyramidal symptoms will be evident. This is also a good time to titrate drug doses and check that the carer is not exhausted.

If the situation is then contained, it is worth reviewing again after 5–7 days for drug side effects, to adjust doses and also to begin to make medium-term plans. At this stage the GP will get sensible feedback from other parties involved in the patient's care such as wider family and CPNs. These discussions tend to continue over the next 4 weeks or so and by 6 weeks some form of resolution about how the patient will be managed has usually been achieved.

What do you put in place to keep situation stable?

GPs will often use rapid intervention services which are set up by bodies such as the commissioning groups or local medical and surgical trusts, and are geared for emergencies as well as being easy for them to access. These teams are focused on providing short-term medical and surgical support. Sadly in the authors' experience, they rarely interact with the mental health services teams either during the emergency or afterwards. This seems to be a result of historic divides between services. For example, district nurses tend not to refer a patient to the mental health services. This makes the GP one of the few people who can ensure the right connections have been made with the mental health service team, and if not can make it themselves.

What should the GP tell the family?

If a patient with dementia presents as an emergency for the first time this is more likely to recur than those who present routinely. There are three possible reasons:

i. the nature of the progression of the disease in the brain which is peculiar to that patient;

ii. the environment, particularly the family or care system which stimulates bouts of agitation or distress;

iii. a visceral element which tips the patient into extreme behaviour or agitation, such as recurrent hyponatraemia or low-grade UTIs.

Point i is unavoidable, but if points ii or iii are not addressed the crises will recur. In terms of the emotional environment it is worth offering a family member a chance to talk separately when the dust has settled as this will give the GP clues about management. Family management and physical illness are dealt with in Chapters 2 and 5.

Social emergency

As has been already said, the age group involved in dementia means that a spouse or sibling who also acts as the patient carer may become physically ill, simply stop coping, become depressed or die. The family members of the next generation are likely to be involved in work, family and other social demands that make prolonged support impossible beyond the first 24–48 hours. This means although there is no intrinsic change in the patient's dementia, they will immediately be in need of emergency care or placement. The difficulties of this situation will be compounded by the fact that the patient will suffer not only from the loss of a familiar carer and concern for that person, but also from the impact of being cared for by unknown people, possibly in unfamiliar surroundings. These factors may result in distress, agitation and behaviour disturbance. For this reason it is worth prompting a spouse or more likely a member of the younger generation to think ahead about possible places for their parent with dementia should the healthier parent suddenly be unavailable. Relatives can think ahead about 'emergency cover' including rotas with family members and any existing social care already in place. Many families imagine they will absorb this care themselves but in reality this is not an option for long periods.

Familiarising the patient with dementia with local day centres and specialised respite centres is another way of planning ahead. These might then be able to offer a temporary daytime support during a relative's hours of work. Some may even arrange specialised home visiting care if a crisis arises. The new larger regional Alzheimer's Society coordinating centres typically cover all these resources. However it must be said they cannot often offer 24-hour or night-time emergency step-up care, unless a special response team structure has been negotiated with the NHS or social services locally.

Local residential or nursing homes often have an empty room and can provide urgent private respite care. It is usually the larger homes or the higher-cost ones that offer greatest opportunity for sudden respite admissions, as they have economies of scale. The issue of respite care mutating into permanent care is a concern for carers and families who see this as betrayal. A GP who has watched and cared for a dementia patient and a suffering spouse over 5 or 6 years is well placed to forestall such agonising, by reassuring the stressed relatives that such a step change in their parents' care is normal and typical in this illness. Emphasising that the respite care is an opportunity to 'try out' a residential home assists the process. The knowledge about what the patient did and didn't like about their respite setting and how and whether it made them 'worse', can then be employed in finding and preparing a patient for a more permanent future placement.

Although GPs are not likely to recommend homes themselves, distressed families appreciate a steer from their trusted doctor.

GP frustrations: best practice vs. worst practice

'Something must be done': the GP at coalface, the family want urgent intervention but the mental health service team says they will visit in 3 days

This is a common and difficult situation. The most common area of breakdown in communication is when the GP asks a non-medical member of the MHSOP team for an urgent review, and this person talks with the family. A referral is more likely to be accelerated if the GP speaks directly with the consultant.

All too often if there is a delay the situation is fudged through a combination of family intervention and intermittent GP input until the MHSOP team arrives.

How does a GP walk away from situation which is unresolved and may also look unsafe?

This is linked to the above. Dangerous behaviour is hard enough to predict in the contained world of forensic science, it is almost impossible to predict in dementia. Families need to be able to tolerate the risk that the patient might roam or encounter other dangers. Therefore it is worth checking where the family are on a scale of understanding this risk, as those who do not will need far more support than those who do. This might appear to be an unsatisfactory approach but the leadership of the GP will help the situation. Reassurance in the form of a promised repeat visit, and contact phone numbers will all help. A confidential anonymised discussion with local community police force or casualty consultant may be prudent. This is pertinent in rural areas if the GP feels the patient might roam or in cases where the family might call an ambulance as soon as they have left. There are now tracking devices and tracking programmes for mobile phones which can be secreted in patients' outdoor coats.

The 'refer to team' seems to be lost in the ether and the GP doesn't know by whom, where or when the patient will be sorted out

This is a common complaint amongst GPs, particularly in those areas of the country where systems have been reformed but are not bedded in and they find it difficult to contact the most appropriate team. During working hours a member of the local elderly mental health services team such as a CPN or a psychiatrist may agree to attend an emergency with the GP. Ideally GPs should also be able to contact the local consultant Old Age Psychiatrist directly for advice. For pragmatic reasons GPs do increasingly develop personal contacts with consultants in Old Age Psychiatry and, where the services are inadequate, it is perfectly appropriate to ask for a direct mobile phone number to a named team member. The structure and use of the multidisciplinary team is discussed in more detail in Chapter 7.

Time delay and poor communication

This is a common problem from within the multidisciplinary teams just as it is between the team and the GP. One major problem is that the teams use forms to communicate rather than real-time conversations, meaning the quality of information sent to the GP is dependent on the ability of the form-filler.

Furthermore teams use the excuse that GPs are busy in their surgeries so it is worth those many GPs who do take calls ensuring that care teams have details of their availability. Sending these in writing to the medical member or key worker of the team removes any opportunity for inaction while opening the channel for effective communication and placing the onus on the care team to engage properly.

Key points

- First presentations of dementia as an emergency are rare.
- The signs of undiagnosed dementia are often in the patient's surroundings.
- Once acute confusion is excluded GPs have time to make a positive diagnosis of dementia even in the face of toxic symptoms.
- Many drug treatments should be given at reduced adult dosage in dementia by cutting tablets.
- Risperidone is the only antipsychotic licensed for use in behavioural and psychological symptoms of dementia, but has elevated risk of ischaemic brain events.
- Ask carers to report neurological side effects when prescribing antipsychotic drugs.
- There are useful, strategic times to review a patient post-emergency.
- GPs' frustration with the current referral and support systems are very well founded but some hurdles can be overcome.

Chapter 5 **Managing families**

No patient with dementia can be treated in isolation. This may seem like a bold statement but by this we mean that the structure surrounding a patient with dementia is as vital to their management as the illness itself. Furthermore any doctor who attempts to manage a dementia patient without understanding the family dynamics which surround them will be hampered in their attempts to the detriment of everyone concerned.

All GPs will understand that family dynamics are complex. In patients with dementia who have often been married for decades to the same person or may have had numerous spouses with a combination of children, stepchildren, grandchildren and even great-grandchildren, these already complex dynamics will be further altered by the disease. In some cases doctors can utilise healthy families to improve patient care, but quite often, doctors will need to help carers to alter the dynamics and free themselves from dysfunctional relationships which have become unsustainable as a result of the disease. By giving partners permission to change the status quo, particularly in the face of a resistant and strong-willed patient, doctors will in turn ensure that the same patient receives the most appropriate care. The authors have gained considerable experience in family work through decades of managing dementia patients and cannot stress enough how important it is for GPs and other specialists to understand the unique influence the condition will have. Only by doing this can doctors hope to improve both the patients' quality of life throughout their disease but also their management in the inevitable terminal stages as well as the legacy which is left behind. In this chapter we highlight some common effects dementia has on families through genuine case histories, and the consequences of the specific interventions by the GPs and specialists involved. As with all the case histories in this book, these cases

---

How to Manage Dementia in General Practice, First Edition. Nicholas Clarke, Farine Clarke, and Denzil Edwards.
© 2013 John Wiley & Sons Ltd. Published 2013 by John Wiley & Sons, Ltd.

have been anonymised to protect those concerned but the principal lessons remain. Clearly the chapter cannot cover the infinite configurations which occur in families, but it highlights examples from the authors' experience, which make the key points about the impact of doctors' interventions in certain family types.

The issue of capacity is also discussed in detail in Chapter 7, as this invariably becomes a subject which everyone managing the patient needs to understand in order to make the correct legal decisions, sometimes against the wishes of forceful families with vested interests.

Mr Castle brought his 65-year-old wife to see their GP, Dr Adams, because she was 'behaving out of character'. The couple had a strong social circle of friends but Mr Castle said his wife had become so rude that they were drifting away. Furthermore her emotional responses were increasingly inappropriate and when the much loved family dog was put down she simply sat at the kitchen table grinning while the rest of the family wept.

On examining Mrs Castle, Dr Adams noted her fatuous affect and thought she might have some frontal damage to explain her behaviour. He referred her to an Old Age Psychiatrist for further assessment and asked Mr Castle to stay in touch so he could receive support.

Mr Castle had been a commercial pilot and had an extremely practical approach to life. While his wife's diagnosis was being established he took all their affairs under his wing from the household chores such as cooking to looking after her horses and chickens. He also made sure she took her drugs and liaised with the hospital team on a daily basis.

Likewise, their 35-year-old daughter, Caroline, gave up her high-flying business career to launch herself full time into understanding her mother's illness. She read all the research she could on the disease and started a local support group, to which she invited medical and nursing specialists to come and speak.

Over the next few years, as Mrs Castle's condition followed an inexorable decline, both the GP and psychiatrist became increasingly concerned about her husband and daughter. The specialist also noted Caroline's desperation to find solutions.

At the same time Dr Adams wondered if Mr Castle was depressed, as his ability to maintain an orderly household became increasingly undermined. Intellectually he understood his wife's illness, but also complained that she refused to keep food in her mouth, used the waste bin instead of the lavatory on purpose and was deliberately aggressive. At the end of the consultation he would always apologise with: 'I'm sorry, Dr Adams. I know it's not her fault. No I don't need any help, thank you.'

Dr Adams and the psychiatrist consulted together and decided to adopt a two-layered approach to manage the family. Their aim was to keep Mrs Castle at home for as long as possible but with sufficient support to ensure Mr Castle didn't become ill or exhausted himself, while at the same time helping Caroline to remain engaged. They also aimed to increase the level of professional support in line with the family needs until the very private Mr Castle might accept a live-in carer.

Dr Adams had a frank consultation with Mr Castle and talked him through the natural progression of the disease, together with practical help which could be made available at any stage. Mr Castle assimilated this information quickly and was thankful, saying that the fear of not knowing what would happen next was actually worse than facing the most difficult scenarios.

Dr Adams gave Mr Castle practical tips on his wife's violence and explained how everyday flashpoints of interference could precipitate attacks. As a result Mr Castle found simple measures, like keeping his wife's buttons loose while dressing her, reduced her outbursts.

By prescribing a hypnotic for Mrs Castle, Dr Adams managed Mr Castle's potential exhaustion by guaranteeing him the 3 nights unbroken sleep a week that he asked for.

Although the Castles had requested out-patient management initially, he now agreed to switch to domiciliary-based support. This meant the district nurses helped to manage Mrs Castle's toileting using diet, fluids and laxatives, together with regular bathroom visits, while reassuring her husband that he need not worry about a 'result'.

The use of the incontinence nurse service and access to incontinence pads via the NHS was also mooted with Mr Castle for the future.

At the same time the psychiatrist provided Caroline with the intellectual and collaborative approach to her mother's illness she needed. He recognised that the support group gave her a sense of purpose and frequently discussed the research findings which she uncovered as she tried to learn more about the disease. They even discussed statins, amyloid immunotherapy phase III UK trials, ezetimibe and heavy metal chelators.

Mrs Castle was treated with acetyl cholinesterase inhibitors and memantine, both alone and in combination at appropriate stages, with good results. The family interventions which Dr Adams and the consultant introduced meant low-dose antipsychotic drugs were needed only for a brief period, when the second-stage crisis 'hit'. The increase in domiciliary care also meant that Mr Castle re-engaged with his friends who provided further support and under-standing once they understood his situation.

The above case demonstrates many aspects of best practice in families of patients with dementia. It shows the different ways in which families will become involved in the disease and also clearly shows how, by actively addressing the family according to their individual needs, the GP, specialist and support teams can deliver maximum benefit for the patient. Taking time to engage the family and support them early on is crucial and will pay dividends in terms of professional time later in the disease and at specific stages where management is more difficult. Sometimes GPs and specialists need to engage other services, such as incontinence nurses, aggressively to ensure they are actively involved. Again, while this takes considerable energy, it is often worth the effort.

In dementia 'family' can mean a number of people. Clearly they can be the spouse, partner or child, but they can also be a same sex live-in companion or close neighbour.

Mr Grange was a proud 70-year-old man with a veneer of inscrutability, which had been cultivated over many years living as an expatriate while working for a large multinational company. He believed that any admission of psychological problems was a sign of weakness and his wife went along with this. When they returned to England and Mr Grange began to have memory problems, the specialist diagnosed Alzheimer's disease. Although he had intermittent insight into his condition, Mr Grange refused to talk about the diagnosis. In turn Mrs Grange found the situation extremely threatening. She went to great pains to maintain a social front and conceal the diagnosis, not only from her friends, but also from her husband.

Things came to a head when Mrs Grange was preparing for a dinner party and her husband read a letter from the specialist. He started to question her while the guests were arriving and she was stuck; unwilling to explain his diagnosis in front of her friends.

The couple had two children with high-flying careers: Carla, who had two young children of her own and to whom Mrs Grange directed most of her anger and frustration, and Duncan, who was left alone by their mother. As a result Carla became increasingly involved in supporting her parents and her job was compromised as a result, while Duncan continued to work without hindrance. Herself stuck and frustrated, Carla complained to her parents' GP, Dr Freeman, and their specialist that they had no business sending a letter which could be found, to her mother. At the same time she forbade them from discussing the issue with her parents. After a telephone conversation with Dr Freeman, the specialist met Carla to talk through her worries. After 15 minutes of indignation she broke down and admitted the stress of the situation and the hurt her mother was inflicting damaged her work and family life.

In turn Dr Freeman consulted with Mrs Grange alone to discuss her main concerns: how to keep Mr Grange's self-respect while allowing her the freedom to see their friends. They discussed how to broach the diagnosis with others and

Dr Freeman stressed she was not being disloyal by admitting to her husband's illness, and the white lies she was telling him were acceptable and understandable. During this consultation, Mrs Grange broke down and confessed that she had been 'horrible' to her daughter but said she was relieved to have 'got everything off her chest' and agreed to regular follow-up for herself.

This case illustrates, once again, the need to understand the family dynamics which play out in dementia care. It also clearly demonstrates that while everyone may be intensely focused on ensuring the patient is protected, the GP, specialists, family and friends can find themselves manoeuvred between 'a rock and a hard place' and subject to collateral damage. Many families feel the need to maintain appearances for the sake of the patient and try to uphold a tissue of lies to achieve this but this situation invariably backfires if it is not addressed early. Doctors have a key role to play in steering families towards healthier outcomes, which is independent of the pure treatment of the patient with dementia.

As in this case, the role of main carer will often fall on the female child rather than the male, even one with equivalent career or family commitments. It is worth GPs and specialists being particularly aware of changes in this family dynamic, because if the supportive relationships become damaged, problems will emerge which eventually impact on the patient. If family members start warring with each other to protect the patient the support networks become even more strained to everyone's detriment.

In this case Dr Freeman and the specialist intervened to address a typical same sex child:parent dynamic which is revealed under stress, namely the diagnosis of Mr Grange's terminal illness. By engaging Mrs Grange and her daughter in a more effective and positive manner the doctors corrected this dysfunctional element so that Mr Grange could continue to be kept at home. Furthermore, once Mrs Grange was able to explain the situation to her friends, they in turn became more supportive and involved, with further benefit for everyone.

Renegotiating the marital contract

Patients who have been married for many years will often have a 'deal' or 'contract' with their spouse which becomes a source of unyielding stress when they become ill. In this circumstance it is perfectly appropriate for doctors to allow the healthy partner to unilaterally renegotiate the contract, typically by telling 'white lies' to the patient. At the same time they should be told to ignore the patient's dysmnesic repetitive postulations or repeated questioning because of their failing memory, like 'water off a duck's back'. However partners will still feel guilty for doing this, which makes the doctor's permission vital.

Mr and Mrs Grange had two key elements to their contract: his need to maintain a social veneer and be in control and hers to enjoy social freedom with like-minded friends. Dr Freeman was perfectly placed to acknowledge these needs while also helping the healthy spouse adapt the contract. He gave Mrs Grange permission to change the contract at an early stage of the disease, when Mr Grange still appeared normal to others, which provided her with considerable relief. It also helped the family to be constructively organised so that Mr Grange could remain at home throughout his illness.

GPs and specialists can also provide the support needed to maintain the key elements of a contract for as long as possible. The key is to focus on the most important parts of the relationship which keeps the marriage 'alive'. Maintaining this makes the dementia patient more real to their spouse as their characteristics are preserved for as long as possible.

In contrast the children may have very little insight into the marital contract and will become confused when the dynamics change. They also need to be supported but cannot actively interfere with their parents' relationship. In the case above, Dr Freeman and the specialist worked out together which parts of the Granges' contract needed to be preserved and focused on doing this. They maintained his self-respect by actively treating him without forcing the diagnosis on him and put in the support which allowed Mrs Grange to remain as principal carer, while also leading an active social life.

By communicating with Carla and David regularly and updating them on their parents' condition, with their consent, the specialist ensured the children did not shoulder all the responsibilities, but were sufficiently involved to not feel guilty.

Emile Emru was a proud Turkish man who had enjoyed a successful but occasionally rocky career running a series of businesses across Turkey and North America. At times his dealings skirted the edge of legality and his companies filed for bankruptcy only to re-emerge in another form a year later.

At the age of 30, he married his children's 18-year-old babysitter, who came from a Turkish village where she had led a simple life surrounded by her family. He remained on good terms with his ex-wife, who lived in England.

Mr Emru's relationship with his children was dominated by three factors:
- *his unreliability and dangerous tendency to take risks which influenced his ability as a provider and homemaker;*
- *his physical harshness and emotionally self-centred approach to life, which was either inherited or learnt from his own father and family culture;*

- *the turbulence which emerged as his young bride began to mature and at the same time separate from him and her own parents – on one occasion she left the marital home for a year and enrolled on a college course.*

Forty years later at the age of 70, Mr Emru developed dementia of mixed aetiology in Turkey. By this time, all four of his sons were both physically and emotionally distant from him, and lived overseas.

In contrast his daughter by his second wife was absolutely devoted to her father and held a childlike, worshipping, affection for him despite being 33.

His second wife had tried for four decades to maintain equal relationships among her stepchildren and her daughter. To some extent she had succeeded as they all liked and trusted her, whatever they felt about her husband.

When Mr Emru started to develop dementia symptoms, his diagnosis was reportedly handled badly in Turkey and the couple muddled along. However, after 3 years, Mrs Emru started to panic and with Mr Emru flew to London where Dr Jack, her husband's ex-wife's GP, agreed to see him. She arrived at the surgery in a state, demanding that 'something must be done urgently'.

Dr Jack had three main challenges:
- *firstly, to establish the correct diagnosis, following a series of mixed and confused investigations and messages from the doctors in Turkey;*
- *secondly, to ascertain the reliability of the history from the couple – this was difficult because of the absence of corroboration by the children and the fact that the patient had deteriorating comprehension;*
- *thirdly, to manage what was clearly a dysfunctional and at times warring family.*

Only by being sure of the above, could Dr Jack be sure of the degree of information, treatment and care the patient himself wanted.

Dr Jack enlisted the help of a specialist Old Age Psychiatrist and together they agreed to base Mr Emru's management from a residential care home on his early life experiences, his culture and the culture of his family.

Once a pattern of care was established, Dr Jack found that children and grandchildren would 'pop up' from around the globe when he visited Mr Emru, to ask him questions. On each occasion he was consistent in his explanations and honest about the diagnosis, management and the inevitable outcome. Over the remaining period, the situation moved from crisis to resolution with a focus on calm, terminal care.

In the last 4 weeks of Mr Emru's life three generations of his family came together as adults for the first time, while he was still conscious and able to reciprocate. At the end, as he lay dying but calm, comfortable and without medication they 'set up camp' in his room. His wife told Dr Jack saying that 10 family members sleeping together in the same room was reminiscent of village life in Turkey and the most natural and dignified ending for them all.

This case illustrates how Dr Jack seized on an unrivalled chance to support the family in a way which helped to manage Mr Emru through the terminal stages of his dementia and also leave a healthy legacy for future generations. By dispensing straightforward, authoritative guidance, while at the same time supporting Mrs Emru in her role of 'head of the clan' and making sense of the family roles, he oversaw a calm resolution to a host of issues.

The GP's key intervention was that he answered all enquiries from this disruptive family in a straightforward and consistent manner. He also respectfully reinforced the appropriate generational boundaries that had been ignored over many years by the patient, who competed with all men, including his sons, and deified all women, including his daughter. Dr Jack treated all the siblings and stepsiblings identically which meant that by the time Mr Emru died the seeds to grow healthy family relationships had been sown.

Two months later Dr Jack received a Christmas card from Turkey signed individually by all five children, their partners and the grandchildren as well as the patient's widow in England, specifically thanking him for his care of the whole family as well as Mr Emru himself.

Complex generational dynamics

At a wider level, this case also shows how stepfamilies with their disrupted age and status sequences and their often jealous sibling to sibling, child to biological parent, and child to stepparent relationships, will pose specific difficulties for doctors managing dementia.

This unique stress for the GP or specialist is matched by an equally unique opportunity to do simple work that revolutionises the family's health, assuming they have the time and capability to do so. Of course dysfunctional families may violently reject any medical intervention, making it wise to be cautious when exploring these dynamics. As in this case, GPs may find it helpful to work with the Old Age Psychiatrists who are increasingly used to dealing with the nuances of generational relationships in dementia, and who in turn may enlist the help of older adult trained psychologists or generic family therapists. Old Age Psychiatrists can be actively involved in meeting and managing the family, or may do so jointly with the GP, or in some cases may simply offer telephone advice without meeting the family. Whatever the route and given their limited time and resources, GPs are well within their rights to request help in this complex but challenging area of dementia care and the authors see this as part of their role as Old Age Psychiatrists.

Mr Sutton was a retired politician who was brought to see Dr Sunil by his wife because she was at the 'end of her tether'.

Mr Sutton had been suffering with memory problems and was given a provisional diagnosis of early Alzheimer's disease by doctors at a clinic in London. However he refused to believe that there was anything wrong with his brain and insisted that his wife took him to a doctor who would give him a second 'better' opinion. He also complained incessantly that the couple should never have moved from their glamorous home in the home counties a few years ago, to deepest Wiltshire where he was 'forced to play golf with rich builders'.

Mr Sutton had been married three times, but was unable to recall the names of his former wives. His present wife was a bright intelligent businesswoman with her own income and two grown-up children with whom she had a close relationship. Her children were extremely supportive of their mother, and, by default, their stepfather. In contrast, Mr Sutton was estranged from his only daughter by his first wife, whom he married when he was just 18, preferring instead his current stepchildren.

Dr Sunil referred the Suttons to the local Old Age Psychiatrist who confirmed the diagnosis of early dementia but also found his inability to recall the name of his former wives demonstrated psychogenic amnesia rather than any complication of his Alzheimer's.

After exploring the nature of the family relationships with the Suttons he devised a management plan with Dr Sunil. The GP consulted with Mrs Sutton regularly to monitor her husband's condition and educate her about the illness, while her children shouldered more of the family responsibilities. They all ensured Mr Sutton was involved in the care of his young grandchildren. Gradually Mrs Sutton changed from feeling desperate and overwhelmed by the prospect of shouldering all the financial, social and caring responsibilities to assuming a higher level of control which reflected her emotional and physical investment in their marriage. Despite Mr Sutton's requests she decided against moving back to the home counties and instead moved 10 miles away to a smaller village house next door to her own son and daughter-in-law. Despite Mr Sutton's opposition to this move it proved to be a success and he went through the gate each day to be with her grandchildren in the shared garden. Mr Sutton was treated with Aricept which improved his disposition and, following a knee operation for his arthritis, he played golf with his wife three times a week. By the same token Mrs Sutton was spared the resentment and exhaustion that would have resulted of any further 'pandering' to his imagined wishes or needs. This change in control took place against a background of his gradually failing capabilities and force of personality due to brain illness, which worked in his wife's favour.

This case illustrates how the threat of trouble to come, rather than a specific change in the patient, is a particular feature of long-term neurodegenerative diseases which can result in carers changing their circumstances inappropri-ately. In this case Mrs Sutton did not move house as her husband mistakenly wished but instead made the right domestic shift under the guidance of her GP and specialist and surrounded herself with greater support to everyone's benefit. If she had moved back to the home counties she might well have become more isolated from her family and Mr Sutton would not have enjoyed family life or watched her grandchildren grow for as long as he did.

Eric Berne's transactional analysis

This case also illustrates how a spouse's ability to maintain strong family bonds with their own children in a divorced setting can be undermined by a needy and isolated partner who does not get on with their own children. An unhelpful dysfunctional pattern of support and care can be established around this needy spouse even before they became ill with dementia.

One model which explains this dynamic was described by the eminent psychiatrist Eric Berne in his transactional analysis 'drama triangle' para-digm. In this all adults move between roles as 'adult', 'parent' and 'child' when relating to others. In the case above, Mr Sutton was already a 'child' who was constantly 'parented' by his wife. The initial diagnosis of a progressive brain disease threw the nature of this dysfunctional relationship into sharp relief. It increased the likelihood that Mr Sutton would remain the centre of atten-tion and neediness, the 'child', despite being relatively well at that stage. The prospect of this made his wife, who was the 'parent' and 'adult', seek help first from a GP then also a specialist. These experts were able to talk to her separately and recognise her own 'childlike' needs as well, which was to be the centre of a loving family and to be cared about. This meant together they could override the patient's self-interest, and allow Mrs Sutton to move back to the heart of her own original family. Of course this not only brought great relief to her, but in turn had a positive impact on Mr Sutton.

It is likely that these roles were always intrinsic to their marriage and probably part of their initial attraction to each other. However, the onset of dementia highlighted the lack of flexibility and the inability to switch roles, which Berne regarded as necessary in a successful long-term relationship.

The only child

Mr House was an 85-year-old retired stockbroker and philatelist whose older wife had died 10 years earlier. His son, Charles, and daughter-in-law, Peggy, were childless and when Mr House developed Alzheimer's the couple provided extensive support. Charles spent much time with his father in a care home but he struggled to settle. When Mr House suffered a syncopal attack which heralded his final decline, the accident and emergency unit sent him to a somewhat sterile new nursing home. Charles worked closely with the specialist and GP to ensure he was cared for appropriately there. When Mr House died 3 months later, his son produced the most beautiful and moving reminiscence album in his father's memory.

This case illustrates the more mutual child:parent relationship typical of an only son who had no need to have children himself and had limited competition for his mother's attention in early life. On the positive side, this son has a depth of understanding of the ailing parent which is uncustomary in a male child. On the negative side, when the parent dies the son may 'lose' a part of himself.

The magnetic compass

Mr Goose was a 90-year-old former army officer with early age-related Alzheimer's disease. He had seen considerable drama during the war, and not only survived extensive bombing together with his men but had also escaped from Colditz. While imprisoned he was supervised by a famous author as part of a university initiative in which messages were sent by the Red Cross parcel service. He remained intellectually active and spoke often of returning to his writing.

Mr Goose was taken to his GP, Dr Hope, by his carer, Jean. Jean complained that Mr Goose had made a pass, not only at her, but also at her mother, which is why she had taken on his care. On examination, Dr Hope found that her patient had mild elevation in mood and was socially disinhibited and referred him to a specialist Old Age Psychiatrist for further assessment. Mr Goose's inappropriate behaviour settled during his brief inpatient assessment where he also received a low-dose atypical antipsychotic and the mood stabiliser sodium valproate.

The specialist met the patient and his two daughters and established that Mr Goose was a narcissistic and demanding man while his daughters had extensive sibling rivalry. Together with Dr Hope he devised a management plan which allowed Mr Goose to remain at home with his carers and gave his daughters some freedom. The latter was the most challenging given their warring state. The sisters competed over their father's illness and insisted on seeing his doctors individually to control his management.

At times Mr Goose's behaviour was dangerous. On one occasion he threatened his carer with a rifle, which was in a locked cabinet, when he thought she was an intruder. When Dr Hope was called she told his daughter to remove this immediately.

Two years later Mr Goose's homecare finally failed and his elder daughter called the specialist in a state of anxiety. He assessed the situation and decided that Mr Goose's combination of disturbed nights, angry outbursts, unsteadiness on his feet, together with his considerable strength, made him impossible for his daughters to manage at home and he needed a specialist dementia care unit. However his eldest daughter felt very threatened by what she considered a failure to look after her father and she broke down. Following reassurance that she had 'done enough' and could do no more but should rather hold fire while the local health teams and his GP determined the best other care option for Mr Goose, she calmed down.

Mr Goose spent his final few months in a residential care home overseen by the specialist and the GP. His daughters came to terms with their own limitations and were able to be with their father at his peaceful death.

This case illustrates a theory that we have come to recognise when treating dementia patients, whereby children without a child of their own do not have the 'selfish magnetic north' of family life, which protects them from a demanding adult parent. Instead the compass needle of care is permanently pointed towards the dying parent. When the specialist explained this theory to Mr Goose's daughters they immediately felt some emotional relief and understood that they had done enough for their father. This in turn enabled them to contain their sibling rivalry and stop trying to be the 'best' at looking after him.

Abused and abusive children

Mr Zimmer was a 95-year-old man with advanced Alzheimer's disease who was admitted urgently to a nursing home when his 92-year-old wife was admitted urgently to a hospital, for what turned out to be alcohol-related disease.

Her son and daughter-in-law, from her first marriage, had left their family home in Wales to look after them but within a few weeks found they were unable to cope and requested the urgent admissions from the Zimmers' GP, Dr Frank.

On arrival Mr Zimmer was found to be unkempt and in poor nutritional health, despite being wealthy. He also showed signs of heavy alcohol abuse, although he was not dependent.

He kept asking why he had been put in a home, and why his step-daughters, whom he disliked, had been allowed to do this. He also wanted to know where his wife was, but did not try to leave or ask to see her.

When Mrs Zimmer was suddenly discharged from hospital she joined her husband in the nursing home where her dominant character and dismissive attitudes to him were immediately apparent. At the same time he became dependent and 'weak' in her presence. When, on an urgent request from the nursing home staff, the Old Age Psychiatrist interviewed her two daughters, he found a mirror image of the Zimmer's pairing: one daughter exhibited a dismissive, angry attitude to her sister who in turn was tearful and inadequate. It became clear that their natural father had died 20 years earlier after an unhappy marriage during which he suffered considerable collateral alcohol-related abuse from his wife.

Mr Zimmer was assessed fully for his dementia and given appropriate advice and treatment in the form of a cholinesterase inhibitor. He began to settle and enjoy the new freedom of the nursing home rather than the one room of squalor he had lived in with his wife. Mrs Zimmer in turn sobered up and although she started to abscond to the pub, the nursing home staff were able to manage her.

The two daughters ignored their stepfather's wishes and sold the family business and other investments as their domineering mother directed, while at the same time showing very little interest in either parent's welfare.

This case illustrates a well known phenomenon, for GPs, namely how abuse, be it financial, emotional or physical, echoes through the generations. In this case the collateral damage is felt far afield by children, their partners, carers and other health professionals.

Different roles in patients with sequential marriages

Some of the cases above highlight the issues which arise in sequential marriages in patients with dementia. The reason to discuss sequential marriages in this book is because dementia is a progressive disease which inevitably involves loss of capacity eventually. In the authors' experience sequential marriages tend to add extra layers of complexity when it comes to managing patients with dementia.

GPs may find themselves having to deal with extra sets of relatives from previous marriages and therefore need to establish from the patient, while they have capacity, whom they wish to involved in their care over future years.

What constitutes a partner?

Because of the typical age of the patients with dementia a trusted partner may not be a spouse, but may take a variety of forms. The authors have seen all of the following: a favourite solicitor or accountant, a life-long secretary or personal assistant, often a long-standing neighbour or a religious companion or the best friend of a now dead only child who becomes a proxy child to the patient. GPs and specialists may deal with any of these partners on behalf of the patient with their consent.

The premature loss of inherited expertise

The older generation typically transfers experience and knowledge to the generation below. This expertise ranges from practical and social skills to religious teaching and psychological and relationship issues.

This is nothing new; for generations, mothers have gone to stay with daughters on the birth of the first grandchild while fathers have offered career advice to their sons anxious to impress the boss at the first meeting. While gender stereotypes have changed over the years, the principle of passing experience on to children and grandchildren remains strong. Learning is also achieved by a mix of didactic advice, modelling, observation, feedback and criticism which is shaped to fit the learner, usually the child or grandchild, in quite specific ways. That this is done by a loving relative gives the process a personal quality which has emotional as well as specific value. In dementia this natural transfer of knowledge is cut short. This is often abrupt while the child is already in shock from the diagnosis. At some levels it is not only prematurely lost, but is also reversed, as the child finds themselves, not only bereft of their teacher but also in the role of carer and supporter. How well children cope with this change will of course depend on many factors, including their level of maturity, which is not always the same as their chronological age, their relationship and experience of their parents and their relationships with other family members. GPs will be fully aware of the problems which can ensue when children find themselves in this position, but this effect that dementia has on the transfer of social capital needs to be understood in order to support families as much as possible.

Key points

- GPs and specialists can ensure the needs of the dementia patient do not undermine the health of the family.
- Eric Berne's transactional analysis theory explains some familial behaviours in cases of dementia.
- The loss of the 'magnetic compass' is a feature of childless children with a dementing parent.
- GPs and specialists are best placed to give partners permission to rewrite the marital contract in patients with dementia.
- Sequential marriage can add extra layers of complexity when managing patients with dementia.
- GPs and specialists must understand the family dynamics to achieve the best outcomes for their patients with dementia.

Chapter 6 **Using the multidisciplinary team**

Dr James was asked to see Mr and Mrs Quinn, aged 85 and 84 respectively, by their daughter who was concerned that her parents were failing to cope at home alone.

When he visited he found it impossible to interview the couple together as they kept interrupting and contradicting each other. If he did manage to separate them the other would immediately reappear and interrupt proceedings again. Their daughter, who only visited occasionally, admitted she was finding it increasingly difficult to have a normal conversation with either parent. She thought her father was confused and her mother was behaving oddly and would disappear for hours at a time, returning late at night.

Mrs Quinn had a history of psychotic illness when she was in her 30s, which necessitated hospital admission and treatment with ECT. She had been taking Parstelin up to 3 weeks before Dr James visited and claimed her supplies had run out. Mr. Quinn had suffered from anxiety which was treated with trifluoperazine for many years.

Dr James contacted the mental health services team for older people to discuss the best way to proceed and it was agreed that two CPNs would visit to interview the couple separately and together.

On initial assessment they decided Mr. Quinn was probably suffering from dementia and, although he was accusing his wife of a number of unlikely things, his daughter said that her mother's behaviour was chaotic. They arranged a follow-up visit, but before this happened Dr Jones was contacted by the police who said the couple were warring at home. Mr Quinn had dialled 999 to say his wife was threatening him with a hammer. At the same time Mrs Quinn accused her husband of assaulting her.

Dr James contacted the mental health services team urgently again and this time two psychiatrists and two CPNs interviewed the couple separately.

How to Manage Dementia in General Practice, First Edition. Nicholas Clarke, Farine Clarke, and Denzil Edwards.
© 2013 John Wiley & Sons Ltd. Published 2013 by John Wiley & Sons, Ltd.

They found that Mrs. Quinn was extremely volatile and irritable, with persecutory delusions about her husband, and concluded that she was probably suffering from a hypomanic or mixed affective disorder. Mr. Quinn had some loss of short-term memory and impaired verbal fluency with obsessional personality traits.

Dr James, the two psychiatrists and CPNs, a case worker and senior case manager from social services together with the Quinn's daughter met together to discuss the couple's management.

The team agreed that separating the couple would be informative and that Mrs Quinn required admission for assessment and to ensure she took her medication. With this aim a psychiatrist and Approved Mental Health Practitioner visited the following day and admitted Mrs. Quinn under the Mental Health Act.

After a week in hospital, Mrs. Quinn remained deluded and hallucinated. When asked why she was there, she said: 'I had a dream that a Roman centurion wanted to marry me and I told my husband and he got angry and sent me here.' She insisted on being addressed as Mrs. Tarquin, and expostulated to staff that she should be allowed to go, as, 'Lord Winston has ordered my release.'

Mrs Quinn also refused to see her daughter when she visited and was so vituperative to her husband on the phone that he declined to visit. She said she wanted nothing to do with him and should be moved to her own flat on discharge. However, following treatment with amisulpiride and sodium valproate her behaviour settled.

Mrs. Quinn had appealed to the Mental Health Tribunal, but she had improved so much and was willing to stay in hospital and take medication, that a discharge plan was compiled to support both her and her husband. Over the following 2 weeks she had an OT assessment of her home, social services put together a care package for Mr Quinn's personal needs, the Alzheimer's Society agreed to supply carers from their Care at Home scheme to keep him company and volunteers from Crossroads also agreed to visit him. Arrangements were also made for Mr Quinn to attend an Alzheimer's Society day centre once a week.

Three months later the couple were managing well at home. Mrs. Quinn showed no signs of mental disturbance and was enjoying life. At the same time, Mr Quinn was perfectly content to let her go out as he now had his own interests. Two CPNs remained in touch, and a healthcare worker helped Mrs. Quinn to keep active.

This case illustrates the difficulty in identifying which member of an elderly couple, who have had a long-term, interdependent relationship, may be suffering from a psychiatric disturbance. In this case, there were grounds for suspecting that either party had a dementing illness, although it was only Mr. Quinn who turned out to have borderline dementia, of vascular aetiology. Mrs. Quinn probably had a symptomatic hypomania which was precipitated by the stress of her husband's condition. He had always been of an obsessive character, but his failing memory made him even more anxious and controlling.

The above case also illustrates the overarching importance of the multi-disciplinary team to provide joined-up thinking, particularly when two elderly patients are living together as is often the case with dementia. This team not only manages the patient with dementia but also helps the carers to cope with acute as well as chronic problems. Furthermore a multidisci-plinary team which works effectively is vital to keep GPs updated about their patients' care both in hospital and when they are discharged home. One of the key aims of the multidisciplinary team is to maintain the patients' quality of life and to ensure they stay at home for as long as possible. Not only is this often far preferable for the patient and their spouse but it can also be more cost effective compared to hospital care.

What in old age psychiatric terms constitutes the multidisciplinary team?

The multidisciplinary team in dementia care usually comprises the specialist Old Age Psychiatrist, community psychiatric nurses, Admiral Nurses, social worker, psychologist and occupational therapist (OT).

Teams may also include a physiotherapist and a speech and language therapist. As in the case above, this team will also dovetail with other wider services which the patient may require including district nurses, social services and the voluntary sector.

The composition of the multidisciplinary team, together with the extent of funding for available services, vary widely across the country, as do the best routes by which GPs can access these. Furthermore the mix of NHS, voluntary sector, social services and private or family input which a patient or their carer might receive also varies enormously from one region to another.

To complicate matters further, the services for the elderly are known by various but equivalent terms in different areas. These include: mental health services for older people (MHSOP) or for the elderly (MHSE), older people's mental health services (OPMHS), community mental health team (CMHT) for older people or for the elderly, as well as other variants.

Which staff are the key points of access for GPs in order of priority?

GPs are increasingly encouraged to refer patients with dementia through a single point of access to the MHSOP. This may be via the local generic mental health services team, who will refer on to the older people's services if warranted.

The access point is often manned by a non-medical person, which means GPs may find this process frustrating, although it is designed to be more straightforward. In this section we discuss the functions of the key team members, so that GPs know who to speak with beyond the single point of entry and also where to concentrate their efforts to forge stronger working relationships.

Clearly the ideal relationship between the GP and the multidisciplinary team is a two-way one in which information moves freely and quickly between the parties. This means everyone involved is up to date and the patients' overall management is well coordinated. We have already discussed the problem of teams communicating with GPs through forms which are dependent on the quality of the form-filler, rather than in real time. This results in justifiable frustration for GPs and one way to mitigate it is to give the mental health services teams contact details in writing, thereby putting the onus on them to provide the GP with telephone updates. GPs are seen as the patient's advocate and the trusted conduit between them and the mental health team and are best placed to translate information and updates on treatment for the family. Patients and families can be suspicious of information or advice from a doctor they have never met before and in stressful circumstances. However they will be far more accepting of this same information if it is imparted by the GP with whom they have a long-standing and trusted relationship.

Even when the family is under some stress and keen for a hospital admission, they are far more likely to contain their anxiety for a GP who says he would prefer to monitor the patient at home and review them in a day or so, than for a relative stranger from the mental health services team. This is particularly true as the person from the team who visits may be different each time.

The duty worker and keyworker

In many areas of the country, the first point of contact for the GP wishing to refer a patient with dementia will be with the member of the old age team who is manning the duty mobile phone that day. At this point the GP may wish to give a range of details including a short medical and psychiatric history and current and past drug treatments. If they have the name and contact details of the patient's friend or relative who is willing to assist coordinating assessment, then it is useful to give these at this stage. If the GP is asked to fill in and fax a detailed form before the referral is accepted they might very reasonably take the view that this an unhelpful barrier and insist on a verbal acceptance, perhaps with an assurance that they will follow up with the paperwork.

GPs should specifically ask when the case will be put forward for the next team allocation meeting and whether anyone will contact the family beforehand to do a preliminary scoping assessment. The latter always reassures the relatives that something is happening. The allocation meetings are usually held weekly and GPs can ask how long the keyworker will take to see the patient. At this stage, GPs are well placed to flag up any difficulties with access or with patient cooperation, together with tips on handling them. The last thing a GP wants to be told is that the case took 5 days to be allocated, the case worker took another 10 days to see the patient and then walked away when told: 'No I don't need any help, thank you' and the case was closed. The simple mantra of 'not taking no for an answer' is a hallmark of a good community healthcare activity around the elderly with dementia.

Community psychiatric nurses (CPNs)

GPs will know that community psychiatric nurses or community mental health nurses are widely available and provide all types of psychiatric care, not just for patients with dementia. Unlike Admiral Nurses, their key focus is on the patient rather than the carer or family.

The rise in elderly patients and those with dementia, means that CPNs are increasingly called upon to manage these patients and their expertise is necessarily increasing. In cases where it is not obvious how far advanced the dementia is, they perform a triage role and will conduct the initial assessments for the memory service. In severe advanced cases, where the diagnosis is obvious and medical treatment is not warranted the CPNs may bypass the memory clinic and enlist social services for personal care or day care, or advise on admission to a care home.

At the other end of the severity spectrum, and especially where symptoms other than those of dementia are prominent, the CPN may arrange an outpatient appointment or visit by the Old Age Psychiatrist. If the patient has mild cognitive symptoms alone, the CPN may perform baseline cognitive testing and either arrange for a follow-up in 6 months or so, or ask the GP to re-refer, depending on local practice.

As well as monitoring drug therapy, CPNs may also provide supportive psychotherapy and cognitive behavioural therapy. Clearly when patients have a coexisting disease such as diabetes, the CPN will monitor glucose control and keep an eye out for infections or any condition which worsen dementia symptoms, although they may also work with district nurses and other community diabetes specialists.

Since the early 2000s some CPNs have undertaken university-based drug prescriber training courses, with the support of their employing trusts and team medical staff. This adds another team member who can prescribe dementia drugs, particularly for the benefit of patients who are restricted to their homes and busy family members who need flexible drug review appointments. Both of the consultant authors supervised the first wave of nurse prescribers in this field and consider them a useful adjunct.

Where CPNs are employed by the local mental health trust, they are based at the local community mental health team headquarters, which may be in a hospital or may be a stand-alone unit in the community. Those employed by the local GP commissioning body are based in GP surgeries. Whichever location, they also act as a point of liaison between the GP and the community, and the hospital-based mental health team. GPs can refer patients with dementia directly to them.

Specialist mental health social workers and care managers for the older adult

GPs frequently say that they are not certain about which element of social services they should access to obtain the best care and support for patients with dementia. This is not surprising because, not only does the depth of available support vary between regions, but also the services themselves seem to be constantly reconfiguring in response to government initiatives and economic pressures.

The National Dementia Strategy, *Living well with dementia: a national dementia strategy* (Department of Health, February 2009), called for joint commissioning of services for dementia patients by health and social services. Many NHS trusts, particularly those providing mental health care, are now officially partnership trusts, structured to support good liaison between health and social care. In practice, the standard and degree of collaboration vary considerably around the country, and do not always reflect the spirit of a partnership. In the authors' experience the care of dementia sufferers tends to be at its most seamless and efficient when there is a social worker with special expertise embedded in the mental health services team. Failing that, liaison improves when the local social services has a specialist team for elderly care. Such teams tend to have good liaison, not only with the mental health services team, but also with local charitable services, domiciliary care agencies and care homes, and are better able to advise on them.

Ideally GPs will know the social worker who specialises in dementia care but, if not, it is worth finding out from the local mental health services team to provide another form of direct access.

Admiral Nurses; an increasingly important part of the mental health services team

Admiral Nurses are senior mental health professionals who specialise in dementia and are appointed by the charity, Dementia UK, to work in this role. They provide care, support and advice for the carers and family of those with dementia. Admiral Nurses perform an important and wide-ranging role and can be particularly useful in carer crisis situations, including exhaustion and depression, and carer conflict, either with the patient, other family members or professionals. They are also helpful in management where the patient has dual pathology and in early-onset dementia where family members may be younger adults or even teenage children.

Admiral Nurses keep independent clinical records and their education and clinical supervision is run by the charity itself at regional centres. They are usually employed by the NHS and attached to the local health services for older people team, although officially partly or wholly funded by the charity.

Some general practices, particularly the larger group surgeries, have Admiral Nurses based in the surgery. This means they are well placed to identify problems with the carers of patients with dementia which is their main role. It also means GPs, who are well aware of the stresses which dementia can have on the whole family, but who also have limited time to monitor this, can be reassured that this important aspect is addressed.

Admiral Nurses in dementia have been likened to Macmillan Nurses in cancer management and their value is emerging in a very similar way. As with many services for those with dementia, availability is still patchy, although numbers are increasing as their role becomes more integral to good care. GPs and relatives can check for availability of Admiral Nurses and access the service directly via the charity website (www.dementiauk.org) and also via Admiral Nursing Direct (number 0845 257 9406).

Other professionals involved in dementia care

Psychologists with specialist skills in areas such as psychometric assessment, individual psychodynamic and developmental theory, behavioural and cognitive therapy, and family work, provide an invaluable resource for a multidisciplinary team in older adult psychiatry. Practitioners may keep records separately, operate their own diaries and caseload quasi independently of the team and benefit from supervision by senior psychologists outside the team and locality. The GP may be able to refer direct to the psychologist in some cases depending on local funding arrangements.

Speech and language therapists and physiotherapists both offer particularly useful services for patients with vascular dementia with coexistent neurological sequelae of focal stroke, such as limb weakness and spasticity, expressive dysphasia and receptive dysphasia. Dementia with Lewy bodies, Parkinson's disease dementia and vascular dementia with vascular parkinsonism also require therapist support with motility and the prevention of flexion contractures, falls and dysphagia due to slowed oesophageal peristalsis. Aspiration can also occur due to vascular bulbar palsy. It is also essential to involve a speech and language therapist soon after diagnosis of frontotemporal lobar dementia to anticipate swallowing difficulties, dysphonia and dysarthria. These can occur fairly early in the illness and at their worst combine to psychologically 'lock in' a patient who remains cognitively sentient with relative preservation of temporal and parietal lobe function. The fear of choking in fronto-temporal lobar dementia with motor neurone disease is a terrifying possibility that will haunt carers and patients unless firm and reassuring guidance is on tap. Some mental health trusts employ these therapy disciplines on a pooled district basis, accepting referrals from any of the locality teams. However this can make access and feedback difficult for a GP.

There is a strong history of occupational therapist involvement in mental health care dating back to the holistic care originally intended within the asylums. This has evolved into OTs having a firm footing in the multidisciplinary teams of community psychiatry and most of all in old age psychiatry. Their original skill base has obvious applications across all the dementias at all stages. This includes home safety and suitability assessments and alterations, including sourcing and installing appropriate bathing aids for frail carers, and identifying the types of social and pleasurable activity most suited to various psychological deficits. Many will now act as generic caseworkers sharing a multidisciplinary team's caseload with the CPNs, and other medical and social care staff on the team.

Once experienced in dementia care for 2 or 3 years any senior practitioner, be they a CPN, social worker, care manager or OT, is likely to be sufficiently skilled in history taking, mental state assessment and cognitive testing to identify dementia patients and separate out those requiring further psychiatric or neuropsychological assessment. They will also be responsible for implementing key-worker type input together with the GP.

Which contact name can the GP give the family?

The patchy availability of NHS care for patients and families, who may have a wide range of medical, home care and social needs, means they may end up with a combination of NHS, voluntary and private input. This is particularly relevant when attempting to ensure the patient can stay in their own home for as long as possible.

For example a patient with dementia may have a package of care comprising their NHS GP and Old Age Psychiatrist with regular visits from the Admiral Nurse and CPN. Individuals may give the family their own contact details. However it may help GPs to discuss names with the multidisciplinary team before giving a list of whom to contact and for what reason, to the family or carer.

Ideally, the care coordinator will be the first point of contact for the patient but if the family have difficulty reaching them consistently then they should be told to find one member of the team in whom they have faith to contact regularly.

The charitable and voluntary sector

GPs and family members share the same access across the voluntary and charitable sector, but GPs sometimes prefer to send patients to the NHS MHSOP team in the first instance. This may be due to a perceived requirement that a local specialist voluntary service wants a definitive diagnosis of dementia before getting involved. Understandably GPs are not always happy to confirm this, particularly in the early stages of the disease.

However it can be helpful for GPs to suggest families make prediagnostic contact with such dementia charitable groups, even before they discuss the condition with the patient. This will help both the voluntary organisation and the family begin to get a sense of the dimension and urgency of need, and how the charity might help, either quickly or in the medium term. At one end of the spectrum a wife might be relieved just to discuss the symptoms of her undiagnosed husband's illness on the phone with an experienced charity caseworker. GPs will be familiar with situations like this, including where a fact-finding spouse might choose not to divulge such a conversation, except perhaps to them in the surgery. At the other end of the scale the local Alzheimer Society centre might offer trained carers to sit with the patient twice a week, while their wife shops. They may also follow with a tactful assessment for a future day centre place, once the patient is in a position to agree to the meeting.

GPs, patients and relatives can access day centres directly in most cases, usually with a simple letter from a doctor or a member of the MHSOP team. Day centres not only provide stimulation for patients with dementia but also give structure to the day and provide much needed respite for carers.

In some cases voluntary and charitable bodies provide services which the NHS has ceased to offer. For example, Crossroads now runs the Dementia Crisis Service in parts of the country. Whilst some organisations are exclusively aimed at dementia sufferers and their carers others have a wider remit. Key charitable organisations in dementia are described below.

The Alzheimer's Society

The Alzheimer's Society is the world's leading dementia charity. It has widespread, although not complete coverage across the UK. The society exists to treat, support and inform those with dementia, not just Alzheimer's Disease, to fund research and to promote the cause of patients through political activity. The Society also runs supportive carer groups and drop-in Dementia Cafés, where information and advice are shared.

The Society's invaluable Care in the Home service is for patients who are unsuitable for day centres, which they also provide, perhaps, because they are at very early stage, or at the severe end-stage of dementia. Care in the Home is manned by paid and volunteer carers with some training and often personal experience who visit patients at home primarily to provide support and respite to carers. Such carers tend to be more skilled at managing patients personally than those from generic care organisations. They will forge strong relationships, so much so that patients may follow them when they leave or become agitated and uncooperative when they are absent.

The role of other charities

Age UK provides day care services not only for those suffering from mild or at the most moderate dementia, but for the frail and isolated elderly in general. Crossroads offers help for carers of patients with a wide range of chronic disabling diseases, such as Parkinson's disease or severe arthritis. They work in close collaboration with local hospices and Macmillan Nurses in end-of-life care.

A list of voluntary organisations together with contact details is given in Box 6.1.

Indirect and direct payments for care at home

Social services accept referrals from the patients themselves or their families, from GPs and from the MHSOP team. GPs may also suggest the patient's power of attorney or main carer approach social services directly to ascertain if they will fund private elements of home care.

Anyone applying to the local authority social services department has the right under section 47 of the NHS & Community Care Act to have an assessment of their needs, and will also have a financial assessment to determine their liability to pay for the services. This is necessary for the application of residential care and at the discretion of the local authority in the case of personal care at home. Local authorities vary greatly in how much they are prepared to pay and at what financial level they will expect individuals to pay for domiciliary care services.

Box 6.1 Voluntary organisations involved in dementia care

- Alzheimer's Society (and Alzheimer International) – www.alzheimers.org.uk;
- Age UK (formerly Age Concern and Help the Aged) – www.ageuk.org.uk;
- Crossroads Care (now merged with the Princess Royal Trust for Carers to form a new body called the Carers' Trust, but still widely known as Crossroads Care) – www.crossroads.org.uk (England, Wales and N. Ireland) www.crossroads-scotland.co.uk (Scotland);
- Parkinson's Disease Society (UK and European) – www.parkinsons.org.uk;
- AgeCare UK – www.agecare.org.uk;
- MS Society – www.mssociety.org.uk;
- Stroke Association – www.stroke.org.uk;
- Carers UK – www.carersuk.org: an umbrella organisation, follow link to local carer support charities.

A social services care manager will assess the patient's needs usually by a one-off home visit and will advise on local carer resources. They will carry out a financial assessment at the same time, to determine what proportion of fees will be paid by the patient. If the client falls below the locally set financial ceilings the care manager will then take the case before their authority's weekly funding panel. Once funding is agreed, the care manager will find carers, organise and supervise them and pay the supplying employer.

Most services are carried out by agencies with which social services usually has a contract. For example, for Meals on Wheels, the company Appetito has virtually country-wide coverage. Other local agencies may provide housekeeping services, such as a weekly cleaner and shopper which the patient usually has to pay for, and personal care such as assistance washing, dressing, feeding and cooking.

Some provide 24-hour live-in care services, but it is rare for social services to fund these, as they are often more expensive than residential placement. Carers, as well as district nurses, perform the vital function of ensuring patients take their medication. Although carers are not allowed to administer this themselves, they can act as reminders and report back if they suspect tablets are not taken.

Some local authorities can assist patients to personalise their package according to their needs, using direct payments, although this facility is relatively rare. Along the same lines, and in an attempt to recognise that everyone is different, various schemes allow patients to tailor their healthcare according to their specific needs and preferences. Sadly these are only available in certain parts of the country and are under increasing pressure when economic circumstances worsen.

Financial ceilings are usually set at nationally agreed levels to avoid immediate disputes and provide the local authorities with some defence against litigation. They represent the savings and assets of any applicant. However, if the patient has a spouse or qualifying dependant sharing the home, that building is typically excluded from the assessment. This means the widowed or those with a spouse already in residential care are far more financially exposed when they themselves come to need state-supported care packages. As a result some patients now arrange transfer of ownership of their property long before such events, to avoid inheritance tax after death and social services deductions before death, putting further fiscal strain on the paying group. A failure of government to increase the thresholds over many years has now effectively enclosed a large proportion of the retired property-owning population within the exposed group. This topic is subject to constant media and parliamentary commentary. At the time of writing, the government has announced plans for legislation to cap the personal contribution to nursing home costs, typical thresholds are given in Box 6.2.

What do home care businesses offer?

As already noted the provision of care for patients with dementia varies widely across the country. Ideally all care would be provided by the state but,

---

Box 6.2 Upper and lower means test limits

Note: these limits may change from year to year

UPPER MEANS TEST LIMITS
England – £23,250
N. Ireland – £23,250
Wales – £23,750
Scotland – £25,250
If you have in excess of the Upper Means Test Limit, including your home (there are certain exceptions to this), then you will be responsible for all your long-term care costs, allowing for any cap on these. If you have below the Lower Means Test Limits, then your costs will be met.

LOWER MEANS TEST LIMITS
England – £14,250
N. Ireland – £14,250
Wales – as per upper limit
Scotland – £15,500

because of the range of needs, this is often not the case. Even those families with relatively low means will end up paying for care in some way. In fact a child giving up work to care for an elderly parent is a form of payment, which is why there has been so much publicity about the need to help carers financially as well as emotionally. GPs will be fully aware that the nature of dementia, coupled with the patient and their spouse's stage in life, will result in a range of needs which cannot be met by one solution. Furthermore these needs are likely to increase as the condition progresses and the patient ages. Although some needs may not appear to be as vital as the dementia itself, in reality they all inter-relate meaning that when one of them is not met the results can be catastrophic.

Similarly, with residential care, there are now few directly managed residential or nursing homes, but local authorities purchase their services, for either long-term or respite care.

Care agencies that provide personal care including help washing, dressing and feeding are more commonly restricted to a single borough or county, although others, such as Saga (formerly Goldsborough), Helping Hands and Consultus, to name a few, have a wider reach. Some local authorities still provide day care, but this is also more usually obtained through voluntary services, or provided by both charitable and commercial care homes.

The role of mobility assistance

Some villages and small towns have volunteer-run mobility services which provide transport for which the patient may have to pay. Some cities provide taxi cards for specific patients, but again this varies considerably between regions.

Local authorities may respond sympathetically to applications for Blue Badge disability parking permits or the equivalent, for those with dementia. This allows their driving spouse or carer to stop as near as possible to shops.

The role of palliative care facilities

Where the patient appears to be in their final weeks or months of illness the GP and family may consider the local hospice. Hospices are increasingly skilled at support in end-stage dementia. Even early in the dementia, the family and patient may find the St Christopher's Hospice end-of-life planning documents a helpful way to start the conversation about the patient's wishes on resuscitation. This is discussed in more detail in Chapter 7 on capacity, and is best undertaken early when the patient is still capable of an informed opinion rather than being left to a late possibly arbitrary decision.

If cancer coincides with dementia, Macmillan Nurses, although not concerned with dementia treatment per se, will find that the presence of the condition has an impact on what they do. They too are likely to welcome early contact from the patient or family.

Key points

- GPs can insist that the multidisciplinary team communicates effectively with them about their patient with dementia.
- GPs should be able to contact named members of the mental health service team.
- Families tend to trust the GPs advice more than that of mental health service professionals.
- GPs provide the conduit between hospital-based teams and the family.
- GPs and carers can contact Admiral Nurses directly.
- Some voluntary bodies have taken on NHS functions in dementia.
- Community psychiatric nurses are becoming increasingly skilled in dementia care.
- Social services provide a range of care which is means tested.
- Some regions allow direct payments and tailored care packages.

Chapter 7 **Capacity, consent and deprivation of liberty**

The diagnosis of dementia does not constitute grounds for assuming the lack of any specific capacity.

Capacity

What does it mean to lack capacity?

The following list, as defined in the Mental Capacity Act (2005) sets out the key principles that must be applied to find a lack of capacity.

- Any assessment is decision and time specific. This means capacity can only relate to one decision at one time.
- It must be due to an impairment or disturbance in the functioning of the mind or brain whether temporary or permanent.
- A person should not be assumed to lack capacity unless all practicable steps have been taken to help him make his own decision.
- There is no absolute measure of capacity but it is evidenced on a balance of probabilities.

For practical purposes, the doctor will usually come to the patient with this information, and then assess whether the following inabilities apply, before determining that a lack of capacity exists to make the decision in question.

- **The inability to perceive and understand the information relevant to the decision.** It is worth noting that a person is not deemed unable to understand the information if he is able to understand this when it is given in an appropriate manner for his circumstances. This includes using simple language, visual aids or any other means.

How to Manage Dementia in General Practice, First Edition. Nicholas Clarke, Farine Clarke, and Denzil Edwards.
© 2013 John Wiley & Sons Ltd. Published 2013 by John Wiley & Sons, Ltd.

- **The inability to remember.** However even if a person is only able to remember information which is relevant to a decision for a very short period, he may still have capacity to make the decision.
- **The inability to use or weigh information.** This is the inability to reach deductive decisions or avoid impulsive decisions in an appropriate setting of understanding. For example a patient may understand an explanation of a medical procedure or a legal document but cannot apply that knowledge. This includes being able to appreciate the reasonably foreseeable consequences of deciding one way or another or of failing to make a decision, despite this being explained.
- **The inability to communicate the decision.** This can be in writing, talking, using sign language or with any other means including using an interpreter.

Why does capacity matter for GPs?

Capacity matters, because any GP or other professional who is managing a patient with dementia will need to decide very early on if they should be talking with the patient about their health, financial and social decisions, or if they should be discussing these with someone else, such as a partner or other representative.

This may seem obvious but it is surprising how often professionals get this wrong and then spend far too much time and energy trying to explain matters to their patients. As with many complex situations deciding at the outset how these will be managed makes for a smoother journey. If changes have to be introduced along the way as the situation alters then doing this against a stable plan also makes things easier.

Under what circumstances are GPs typically asked to assess capacity?

Usually the patient's solicitor asks the GP for advice in the process of preparing or revising a legal document such as a will or power of attorney.

GPs should exercise caution when responding to a solicitor who has been retained and paid for by a patient's relative, or, for that matter, any other party. Again, this seems obvious but enquiries are often presented as an apparently well meaning request for information, with the patient's name in bold at the top of the letter, which implies consent and also that the GP should be a willing ally in protecting their patient's interests. This approach may be entirely proper but can create a false expectation that the question is straightforward and the GP is simply being asked to endorse a position that has already been established. Thus a letter couched in terms such as 'the client would like to make a will, please confirm he has testamentary capacity' or 'the client cannot manage his property and affairs, please complete form COP3' is asking the GP to agree to a premise that has been set by someone else. It is often easier to agree than to disagree.

To assist in such a case, the GP must take care to form his or her own opinion and unless the patient's condition is already well known, start with the presumption that the patient is capable. Thus the first question will be: can the patient consent to the assessment taking place and to the information being released? If the patient lacks capacity then the GP can and should refuse to release information other than to or for the Court of Protection. This might be given to a deputy appointed by the Court to manage the patient's affairs, a Court of Protection Visitor or the Court itself. Where an application to the Court has not yet been made and the patient lacks capacity to give informed consent to its disclosure, the GP may release evidence directly to the Court or to a solicitor on the clear understanding that the information is confidential and subject to legal privilege. Where the request for information comes from the donee of a lasting power of attorney, the donor may still have capacity (as a lasting power of attorney can be created while a person has capacity) and therefore the donor's authority should be sought if it can be obtained. Other than this they are under no obligation whatsoever to release details of their patients' private health matters. The same protection also exists after death.

The number of solicitors who specialise in mental capacity, and other issues affecting older people in particular, is increasing. Many of these will already have a special interest in mental health law and are likely to contact GPs about testamentary capacity, lasting power of attorney and applications to the Court of Protection. GPs will also be consulted about capacity to make decisions involving end-of-life care, also known as 'living wills' or 'advanced directives', as the case below illustrates.

Mrs Drake was a 86-year-old woman who had a very active lifestyle until she developed severe depression which was diagnosed by a consultant Old Age Psychiatrist. Although she used to play bowls three times a week, she lived alone in a large house and was becoming increasingly isolated and less able to manage on her own. Together with her GP and the psychiatrist she agreed to move to a nursing home where she could be better cared for and would enjoy the cama-raderie of like-minded residents.

On admission to the home Mrs Drake was asked to sign a form about CPR at which point she panicked and was unable to deal with the implications of what she was being asked to do.

When she met with her consultant psychiatrist that afternoon she declared that 'of course she wanted CPR'. However over the following weeks, during which he visited regularly to monitor her depressive illness, she repeatedly reiterated that her greatest fear was losing control and being confined to bed and unable to exert her free will.

At the time Mrs Drake was unable to discuss this contradiction between her fears and her agreement to the urgent resuscitation that might bring her back to exactly such a debilitated existence.

After 2 years of psychotherapy and antidepressant treatment, Mrs Drake was asked to consider a more sophisticated document from the nursing home. She discussed this with her psychiatrist and amazed him by weighing up the pros and cons and deciding that she didn't want CPR. By this stage she was physically and mentally healthy and also surrounded by a number of residents who were 10 years her senior but also in good health. Mrs Drake said she now appreciated the health she enjoyed but would not want to prolong her life and risk incapacity. Her loving family and the nurses in the home agreed with her and supported her decision.

This case illustrates an important misconception, which is that the consent or refusal of consent can necessarily be obtained from someone during a quick and straightforward conversation with a doctor. It is really important that all those involved in consent understand that the opposite can be true. Even where the patient appears to have capacity they may hide their true wishes and needs from family, their GP and even from themselves. Underlying issues may emerge slowly during repeated visits by the GP and others involved in the patient's care. In some cases nurses who see the patient often and form closer, less daunting relationships, are best placed to have these conversations. The hospice movement led by St Christopher's Hospice has undertaken extensive work on developing paper support for end-of-life planning for the old or ill, and those who care for them. These documents form a good basis for practice nurses, counsellors, GPs and others to take forward discussions. As well as using their extensive long-standing knowledge of the patient and the family, GPs can facilitate end-of-life discussions concerning diagnosis, prognosis and the merits of available treatments.

How does a GP go about assessing capacity?

For everyone involved in assessing capacity, the following five principles apply.

- **The assumption of capacity.** This may seem obvious but a person must be assumed to have capacity unless it is established that they lack capacity.
- **Help or enable patients to make decisions.** In other words a person should not be assumed unable to make a decision unless all practicable

steps to help them do so have been taken without success. This includes using pictures, diagrams, writing and also the Internet. Even where the patient lacks formal capacity, they should be encouraged to participate in the decision as far as their level of understanding permits.

- **People are allowed to make unwise decisions.** A person should not be treated as unable to make a decision merely because they make an unwise one. There is an exception to this rule which is rarely seen in dementia where the impulsiveness and volatility of a patient's decision removes their ability to make the decision based on understanding. Examples include some learning disabilities or anorexia nervosa.

- **Best interest must govern delegated decisions.** If the decision making is delegated to another person or body because of incapacity, then it must be made on a 'best interest' basis. This means making a best estimate of what the person would have wanted. To do this properly often involves discussing carefully with relatives what the patient would have wanted if they had capacity. The patient's own current wishes and feelings must also be considered to the extent that they can be provided. The following process will help GPs to determine best interest. It might best be summed up in the aphorism 'always put the patient first'.
  - Make a checklist.
  - Weigh each item in the balance.
  - Empower.
  - Consider patient's beliefs and values.
  - Consult others.
  - Do not substitute your own judgement.
  - Protect the patient – your duty of care is to your patient and not to anyone else.

- **Least restrictive approach.** The decisions must result in the least restrictive interventions.

A practical approach to capacity

It may help GPs to approach capacity on the basis that the person responsible for establishing capacity is the person responsible for enacting the decision. For example the solicitor drawing up the will is responsible for determining capacity. The surgeon performing the operation is responsible for establishing capacity. The court may be asked to rule on the evidence but this does not absolve the original person of responsibility. Trusts are increasingly going to the Court of Protection to support their clinical decisions where patients lack capacity.

However, it is sometimes forgotten that it is the doctor and not the judge who wields the scalpel. All the Court can do is permit a procedure to take place if the doctor believes it to be in the patient's clinical best interests. The Court cannot compel a doctor to carry out a particular procedure or demand a treatment for which there is no funding.

The unique skill doctors bring is in their ability to match diagnosis and prognosis with the current measurement of capacity and make sense of it. For example, a GP can say, '*This patient has dementia, he has capacity now but will probably lose it within a certain period of time.*'

Capacity fluctuates. This makes capacity assessment a cross-sectional process which can be repeated at any time. If a patient does not have capacity it is prudent to come back another time and see if they do. A patient may be better in the morning than in the afternoon, or may improve after a course of antibiotics have cleared a urinary tract infection. Often it can take several attempts to complete an assessment. Even the location may affect capacity. A patient may be confused in hospital but more relaxed at home.

All practicable steps should be taken to help a patient make his own decision. It is important to energetically enhance the communication lines, for example by checking the patient can hear and see properly. Is their hearing-aid working? Is the light sufficiently bright? As well as making sure the patient understands the doctor's accent, and that they are calm and have a pen which works. A doctor's skill at putting their patient at ease pays dividends. Some polite social conversation can be a very effective means of providing reassurance as well as measuring capacity. As described in Chapter 1, introductory questions about a patient's home, family, occupation, hobbies or pets are a useful means of measuring memory and attention to detail. A patient who can recite the names and ages of children and grandchildren is more likely to have capacity than one who cannot remember these details.

The doctor can begin asking more specific questions once the ambience is right, but if the patient fails the doctor should be prepared to help with some further information and then reapply the questions. For example the GP might ask the solicitor to sit in the room at the same time and remind the patient about the terms of the will. The doctor can then check the patient understands this, so as to be satisfied as to the correct level of understanding before signing the will. Care needs to be taken to ensure that whilst the patient has the information prompts relevant to the decision, they also have an opportunity to show an understanding of the subject matter. It is not uncommon for legal advisers to spend time reading out or explaining a complex legal document and conclude with a simple question, '*Do you understand?*'

Finally, remember that the more complicated the affairs or the more valuable the estate, then the more likely it is to be contested. For example a will made on the deathbed raises the bar for the level of evidence needed to exclude incapacity.

Testamentary capacity

The following lists the requirements a patient must understand to demonstrate testamentary capacity, together with questions GPs can ask to determine each one. The answers should be recorded verbatim:

* The nature of the act of will making.
  Can you tell me what a will is?
  What will happen to a will once you've signed it? Can you change it? When does it come into effect?
* The effects of making a will in the form proposed.
  What sort of things do you put in a will? Is it better to leave everything you have to one person or institution or to divide it up?
* The extent, not necessarily the value, of the property. GP should look for a comprehensive list appropriate to their patient and gain an understanding of for example whether the patient knows they own the property.
* Understanding and appreciating the claims of all the people to whom they should have regard. This last test is based on reaching some kind of moral judgement between individuals.
  You don't have to tell me who is actually in your will, but what sort of people might you put in a will?
  Do you think there are some people who deserve a larger portion in a will than others?
  Are family ties more important than friendship or repaying good deeds in the past?
  Do you think the needs of the recipient should alter your bequest to them?
  Do you think children and grandchildren should always be treated equally?

The patient should be aware not only of who is included in the will, but also the consequences of failing to make a will (intestacy) which may unintentionally exclude some intended beneficiaries. Amongst these people may be those who lack any obvious claim where there is no will, or the beneficiaries under an existing will. Thus an assessment of testamentary capacity may require information about an earlier will.

The following questions act as a scoping exercise for doctors who are best placed to detect fraud. Patients are frequently able to explain why they may leave money to their gardener and not to their doctor and large bequests to professionals should raise a warning flag.

Would it be appropriate to put the following in your will: a policeman, milkman, postman, gardener, cleaner, solicitor or your doctor?

Patients will typically leave bequests to a trusted long-standing gardener or cleaner or postman, not the solicitor or the doctor. Although GPs may feel awkward asking this question and never seek bequests themselves, it is wise to know in advance how a patient thinks.

Lasting power of attorney

There are two types of lasting power of attorney: one for property and affairs and one for health and welfare. This replaced the enduring power of attorney which, provided it was executed correctly prior to 1 October 2007, is still valid.

To assess capacity for a lasting power of attorney for property and affairs, the patient must satisfy four basic requirements of understanding:

- that the attorney will assume complete authority over their affairs and subject to any restrictions in the power the attorney will be able to do anything with the property which the donor could have done;
- any decisions made by the attorney where the donor lacks capacity must be made in the donor's best interests;
- the authority will only come into effect when the lasting power of attorney has been registered by the Public Guardian, irrespective of the donor's capacity;
- the authority can be revoked at any time although the Public Guardian will have to be notified to cancel registration.

Where a lasting power of attorney for personal welfare matters is concerned, the patient needs to understand that it will only be effective in respect of those decisions which the donor lacks capacity to make.

The following questions GPs may ask apply to both types of the lasting power of attorney.

Do you know what a power of attorney is?

Do you know what it gives someone power to do?

What sort of areas of your life or possessions might it give power over?

What sort of people might be suitable for you to give such power to?

How long do you think such a power would last?

Do you know the difference between a regular power of attorney and this different type of lasting power of attorney? The difference being that regular power of attorney is a temporary measure which can be revoked by the donor at any time and is automatically invalid should the donor lose capacity.

At this last question even well informed patients may hesitate and will need explanations by the GP or lawyer. Once this is given, they can be retested.

Within the Mental Capacity Act (2005) a detailed form, COP3, now exists for completion when a patient lacks capacity.

Consent

Capacity to consent to medical procedures

GPs are familiar with the spirit and methodology governing patient consent including the central principle that no one can consent to an operation other than the patient themselves. With patients who lack capacity, all a court can do is permit a procedure to take place if the doctor believes it to be in the patient's clinical best interests. If the patient lacks capacity, then any decision must be based on the components of best interests for the patient as given above.

What should GPs do if the family disagrees?

GPs will often rely on the family to understand a patient's wishes, beliefs and values. In the authors' experience, simply saying to a patient's daughter, '*You cannot make the decision for your mum and neither can I. What is important is that we jointly understand what your mum would have wanted in this situation if she'd been asked 20 years ago. That is not the same as what you would want to happen to you*,' immediately engages the family in helping to make the right decision. This approach also gives them some relief from the burden of the decision. The need to separate their own preference from that of their relative is important. One interesting study, published in the BMJ (1996), showed that 83% of relatives of patients with Alzheimer's feel they should not be told the diagnosis as it would distress them. However when it came to themselves 71% said that they should be told. Is this cognitive dissonance or hypocrisy?

With a reasonable family, this approach normally results in an accord between the GP and the family.

In cases where the family disagrees with the GP's conclusion, provided the doctor has conducted their assessment in a robust, repeatable manner as described which will stand up in court, they should adhere to their decision. This highlights the importance of following the correct processes, using every means to ensure the patient is settled during testing, using explanation where necessary and also recording all answers verbatim. Not doing so results in problems, as illustrated in the case below.

Mr Craig, a retired 70-year-old man went to see his new GP, Dr Ford, after he discovered that his 50-year-old professional daughter had registered his enduring power of attorney several years before with the Court of Protection.

Mr Craig had moved into a large house on a road the locals dubbed 'Millionaire's Row' some 3 years earlier.

Dr Ford looked through the notes and could only find a single episode of possible confusion following a brief period where Mr Craig's previous GP prescribed temazepam.

After an initial examination which did not reveal any abnormalities, Dr Ford referred Mr Craig to the Old Age Psychiatrist. The specialist found Mr Craig to be very eloquent and able, despite having amnestic type mild cognitive impairment. Mr Craig also had remarkable practical abilities and indulged his hobby of restoring vintage aeroplanes, which he then gave to local aeronautical museums. His only complaint was slight forgetfulness since he crashed a car at a rally some 5 years previously.

Based on these findings, the specialist told Mr Craig's solicitor that the patient was able to satisfy all the components of an assessment of capacity to complete a lasting power of attorney and also a more general ability to manage his affairs. He gave a polished, near legal description that satisfied testamentary capacity.

Mr Craig moved in with his younger sister for comfort and there followed vigorous opposition by his daughter who made unsolicited calls to the specialist and solicitor. She also turned up at her aunt's house, unannounced but accompanied by a solicitor.

Her main objection was that her father wished to give some money and a small proportion of his savings and pension, to her, but did not want to sell his home. Mr Craig told Dr Ford that he did not want to disinherit his daughter but also wanted, 'To stay in control of my affairs until I am no longer reasonably able to. I don't want her to run my life.'

Based on the GP and specialist findings, application was then made to the Court of Protection for a decision to reverse the enduring power of attorney and this was duly confirmed after 3 months. The patient resumed control of his affairs. After taking further advice the patient rescinded his previous enduring power of attorney and completed a new one in which he named an older and younger solicitor as independent attorneys. He also made minor alterations in a new will. These new documents were countersigned by the specialist, after a detailed and contemporary review of Mr Craig's mood, mental state, cognition and specific capacity for those tasks. This was done during an hour long, one-to-one consultation. Furthermore, the solicitor acted as a co-signatory. Again this was only done once the specialist confirmed that the nature of the tasks described by the patient matched that described by the solicitor who was responsible for enacting the decisions.

This level of care was necessary because of previous litigation, the value and complexity of the holdings and the anticipated likelihood of further challenges both before and after death. Two years after this episode the patient continued to show no significant cognitive deterioration, and was enjoying living with his younger sister.

Will GPs ever be called to give evidence about capacity and how should they approach this?

Currently, in the UK the courts tend to rule on disputed matters, such as those concerning marital wealth and finance, rather than other aspects of an individual's circumstances in dementia. As such, they tend not to ask doctors for an opinion about capacity where it relates to social matters.

Deprivation of liberty

What is meant by deprivation of liberty?

The Mental Capacity Act (2005) was introduced to give statutory protection to those who lacked capacity or were confused. This is because, despite planned changes to the Mental Health Act (1983 amended 2007), patients who had been retained in hospital lacked legal recourse to challenge their detention. If, for example, such patients were admitted to hospital informally rather than under a Section of the Mental Health Act, there was no provision for appeal if they or their family opposed the admission. This became known as the 'Bournewood gap' after the case of an in-patient with learning disability who lacked capacity, against a Health Authority of that name. The European Court at Strasbourg found that his continued informal in-patient care, whilst disregarding his protests, was unlawful.

These safeguards were put into place to ensure hospitals and residential care and nursing homes only restrict a patient's liberty when there is no other way to take care of them safely. They apply to patients with dementia who are informally admitted to a care home and are deprived of their liberty, when they do not have the mental capacity to make the decision about their care or treatment. They also ensure any deprivation is done correctly.

Why does it matter for GPs?

Very occasionally, GPs will be approached by social services or managers of NHS care homes and often distant relatives with concerns that there is undue restriction on the patient's choices.

How can GPs pick up deprivation of liberty?

Surprisingly there is no formal definition of the deprivation of liberty. This means GPs and others involved in a patient's care will have to judge whether or not a restriction on their freedom is appropriate and proportional for them. At a formal level, cases which have been defined as a deprivation of liberty include:

- restraining a patient in order to bring them into hospital;
- giving medication against a patient's will;
- staff taking all decisions about a patient including choices about assessments, treatment and visitors;
- staff refusing to discharge a person to others or restricting access to their family or friends
- However, repeated attempts by a patient to leave do not justify deprivation of liberty safeguards in themselves, if repeated reassurance and discussion successfully distracts or terminates the apparent desire to do so. Also,

locked doors are not necessarily a deprivation of liberty if there is a route or pathway by which a patient can leave. They should either know about this already, be told about it, or be able to ask staff about it.

What duties do GPs have towards their patients about deprivation of liberty?

Should a GP have reason to believe that a patient is being deprived of their liberty but that they have capacity and the staff insist there is no problem, they will rightly need to resolve the issue. Ideally the care staff will engage with the GP to ensure the patient has a means of redress, such as being able to leave with staff. However, if they do not then the GP is right to inform the Deprivation of Liberty Office, who will undertake an assessment for Deprivation of Liberty Safeguards.

If a GP feels a patient in a residential home is subject to deprivation of liberty and this is justified, they should also check that a Deprivation of Liberty Certificate is in place. It is against the law to deprive a patient of their liberty without an 'authorisation' to do so in place for that patient. Managers of care homes have to apply for such authorisation for every patient and this is made in writing to a supervisory body. In an emergency the management can grant itself urgent authorisation lasting for 7 days at the same time as applying for standard authorisation. This lasts for a maximum of 12 months before it must be renewed.

If the GP feels deprivation of liberty is not justified, they can ask social services to appoint an independent mental capacity advocate (IMCA) to review any previous assessment or authorisation. However despite their creation in law 7 years ago, IMCAs are rare and far fewer have been appointed than intended. This may be because their role is solely in information gathering, rather than creating or advocating a new plan.

In contrast, the right of independent mental health advocates (IMHAs) to copy and share relevant parts of the medical or social services files with the sectioned in-patient they represent, has been keenly taken up. Many thousands of detained patients with capacity have been assisted by IMHAs who are often fellow in-patients.

What if the family disagrees?

Once a patient has lost capacity, GPs may find themselves pushed in the opposite direction to the spirit of the Mental Capacity Act because carers and relatives want the patient to be contained 'for their own good'. This is because their greatest fear is the patient wandering off and doing themselves damage.

In our experience, a family which resists or resents the apparent deprivation of liberty of a patient is of particular importance in weighing up the likelihood of deprivation because they know the patient well and sense something is very wrong. As already stated, in reality, the vast majority of families object if doors are NOT locked on their demented relatives who wander, rather than the other way around.

Mr Carpenter was a 79-year-old former bricklayer who came from an impoverished inner city background and left school at 14 to start manual work. In contrast his son, David, attended the local grammar school, then Oxford University and became a partner at a successful law firm. David soon moved his parents into his luxurious gated house in London where the family lived in comfort. However, when Mrs Carpenter died after 60 years of marriage, her husband was left rudderless. At about the same he started to become confused and David asked his GP, Dr Crick, to see him. After a thorough assessment she concluded his memory and orientation problems were typical early symptoms of a late age dementia but agreed with David that these were not severe enough to interfere with his relatively independent life on the estate.

However, as the illness progressed Mr Carpenter began to try to leave the gated compound by forcing the gates or even climbing them, while insisting that it was not his proper home. This is a relatively common belief in patients with dementia.

David and his sister Jayne decided to move their father to a very luxurious older living community 800 yards from the house, rather than a dementia care unit believing that he was 'too well for that'. A form of subdued chaos followed, during which Mr Carpenter became increasingly distressed and restless, and even threatened staff with physical violence. His main desire was to 'get out and go home'.

At this stage Dr Crick asked the Old Age Psychiatrist to review Mr Carpenter and together they agreed to a trial of sertraline and low-dose diazepam to reduce irritability and calm him down. However because this had limited effect they also tried other anxiety-reducing drugs together with explanatory discussions with Mr Carpenter and his relatives. The manager at the home decided to lock the doors of the unit, which had previously allowed a steady stream of visitors to enter and leave. Although Mr Carpenter would not try to run away while on his 2-hour accompanied walks to the local village, he would try to break out of the locked doors. He would also comment on the free 'comings and goings at the home' by other residents.

Both Dr Crick and the Old Age Psychiatrist were concerned that the use of medication, the use of a locked door, albeit with free passage on request, and the collective 'ignoring' of Mr Carpenter's desire to be somewhere else all represented the deprivation of his liberty. His family did not share this concern, typically wanting more reassurances that he was safely contained from harming himself in some way. The Care Quality Commission were asked for their advice and after consideration approved his continued residence whilst a full assessment was made together with attempts to alter the elements of deprivation.

The day after this decision, Mr Carpenter eluded his observers and began to walk to London on the hard shoulder of a nearby motorway, possibly aiming for his original childhood home. The police brought him back. Two days later they again observed him on the motorway shoulder apparently unaware of the inappropriateness of his position. This time the specialist reviewed Mr Carpenter and decided that he did appreciate the danger of lorries passing, and that there may even have been an element of 'choice' about his alarming route. He commented that it is unusual for patients with dementia, even in advanced stages, to lose all road sense although they may not necessarily know the direction that they are going in, so called topographical agnosia. They tend to maintain a relatively safe wandering ability in civilised surroundings, and this may have explained why Mr Carpenter did not try to cross the motorway lanes.

Eventually Mr Carpenter moved into his daughter Jayne's house with a live-in carer, whom he liked. His desire to be elsewhere was greatly reduced and he was far more accepting of the locked front door.

This case represents an example of a GP becoming involved in apparent deprivation of liberty. Deprivation of liberty is not straightforward. Restriction of liberty is acceptable in law but the challenge is in understanding at what point this restriction tips into deprivation. The fact that these safeguards have not been used as frequently as anticipated by those who compiled the Mental Capacity Act, illustrates this difficulty.

Therefore the best advice for GPs who do become involved is as follows.

- First of all assess if the capacity is indeed missing. In Mr Carpenter's case he retained remarkable conversational and memory abilities, despite his mild dementia. This made it difficult for the admitting home to conclude that he lacked capacity to decide where he wished to live. This was true even at more subtle levels. However once he had returned to the motorway, despite explanations and requests not to, it became harder for the family and care home staff to argue with the GP and specialist that he retained capacity to fully understand where he might live and how he might get there. This meant the home had to act within the Mental Capacity Act to unlock the door and discharge the patient, or to obtain a Deprivation of Liberty Safeguard Certificate. In this circumstance, the borderline incapacity of the patient, the unsuitability of the unit for safe restriction of movement, and the unwillingness of the family to see him moved to a dementia care unit with a locked door, resulted in discharge. One might argue that this is exactly the type of protection envisaged by the authors of the Mental Capacity Act (2005). It did not allow the informal containment of the patient to continue.

- Are there actual physical or psychological mechanisms in place which result in deprivation of liberty? In this case, if we assume Mr Carpenter lacked the relevant capacity, the locked doors, sedative drugs and a one-to-one companion discouraging him from leaving all represent a deprivation of liberty.
- Is there a potential redress for the patient from the deprivation of liberty? In Mr Carpenter's case this was partial: he did not possess a key to the door himself but was able to ask the carers to accompany him out each day for hours at a time. He did not refuse medication but would have been allowed to, although he may not have completely understood the loss of beneficial effects at all times. At times he may have viewed his companion as a boon rather than an imposition.

In this case, the GP was also instrumental in managing the changing situation to a new one which is both safe for the patient and his carers, and keeps within the bounds of the law. Mr Carpenter's move out of a care home took him out of the ambit of the Mental Capacity Act (2005) Deprivation of Liberty Safeguards. The GP and specialist then supported his settling in, by checking that the patient wished to be there on an ongoing basis, and prescribing suitable medication for a new live-in carer to manage. They also supported the family where he then resided. Part of this support was talking through alternative future care pathways that would ultimately progress to a trial placement at a specialist dementia unit care, once all had agreed the time was right.

Key points

- The diagnosis of dementia should not assume a lack of a specific capacity.
- A GP's assessment of capacity, including testamentary capacity, should be robust, repeatable and stand up to legal scrutiny.
- Capacity fluctuates and assessments should be repeated if necessary.
- Patients should be coached to ensure they understand questions when their capacity is assessed.
- GPs are well placed to ensure deprivation of liberty safeguards are in place.
- The patient's advocate must be aware that families rarely complain about deprivation of liberty.

Reference

Maguire, C.P., Kirby, M., Coen. R. *et al.* (1996) Family members' attitudes toward telling the patient with Alzheimer's disease their diagnosis. *British Medical Journal,* **313**, 529.

Chapter 8 **Choosing a residential home**

GPs are often asked by families of patients with advanced dementia how to choose a residential home or if they can advise them on a particular one. It is worth taking some care here and, in our experience, best to avoid the temptation to offer insights such as: '*I would not put my own mother in that home.*' While this may be absolutely true for the GP concerned, it is an obvious denigration of the home which may come back to haunt them should word get out. The owners may accuse them of unprofessional behaviour or, worse, sue the GP for defamation. Relatives talk to neighbours and friends in the community, often asking each other the same questions and it is more likely for a GP's well meant but inflammatory comments will be passed on. Of course if any doctor feels very strongly about a particular home and has evidence to support their concerns then they should certainly make those feelings known to the appropriate authorities and will be taken seriously.

Having said this, GPs will have sound and valid views about the strengths and weaknesses of one particular home versus another in their region, which they should be able to talk about with relatives. In these discussions it is more positive and less hazardous to highlight the beneficial qualities of a particular home and relate these to its suitability for the patient.

The authors would like to believe that social services use their influence to improve the quality of care homes by listing them as 'approved'. However they can also blacklist homes which they consider to be too expensive with the aim of keeping costs down. Failure to list and fund acts as effective blackballing of excellent homes. This is done under the guise of saving taxpayers' money.

All homes are subject to inspection by the Care Quality Commission (CQC). Prospective residents and their families can find more details about

How to Manage Dementia in General Practice, First Edition. Nicholas Clarke, Farine Clarke, and Denzil Edwards.
© 2013 John Wiley & Sons Ltd. Published 2013 by John Wiley & Sons, Ltd.

the home on their website. These details are factual, and pay attention to how well a home fulfils the Commission's criteria which tend to be operational and well defined, but do not give an aesthetic feel for the home.

Is there a difference between homes?

There are a variety of homes available which fall into a range of categories, but the following broad descriptions may be useful.

- A dwindling number of homes are managed and financed by Social Services from central funding. They charge low fees and include some specialist experimental projects, such as the Domus Project of southeast London which set out to improve care in deprived urban environments.
- Small private homes: these are family run or small business residential and nursing homes for older people. They may appear to be outdated, or not 'cutting edge' but at the same time offer the type of old-fashioned, personal care that is attractive to a generation which is used to that approach. Some of these homes form themselves into associations for mutual support, staff training and enhanced market clout. Seeing people sitting in a circle is not common nowadays, but that does not mean it is not suitable for some older people. Of more concern is seeing a patient suffering benign neglect from overworked staff in a so called executive single room.
- Homes that are not strictly speaking residences for dementia patients can nevertheless give sanctuary and care to many people with the disease, even in advanced stages. They usually will not accept as residents people who are already suffering from dementia but in the authors' experience will usually continue to care for those who arrive as 'frail elderly' and develop dementia during the course of their stay. This recognises the reality of dementia in older people who may have been in a residence for several years, and is the more humane approach.
- Senior living environments: the last decade has seen an expansion of not-for-profit and commercial property development which provides a combination of senior living environments, theoretically for those without dementia, together with an attached unit to manage those with obvious disease. This arrangement means older patients can be transferred between the two units when needed. Typical homes within this sector include the Barchester and Sunrise organisations.

What support or activities should be intrinsic to a residential home?

One man's peace and quiet is another woman's boredom and the type of home selected by patients will vary depending on a host of variables including proximity, style and the available activities. One of the most useful facts GPs can tell families, who tend to look at the other residents when visiting homes, is that, on the whole, the principal friendships the patient forms are with the members of staff, not with the other residents. Staff tend to be younger, more energetic and more likely to enjoy extended conversation. Furthermore, the average occupancy time of a patient with advanced Alzheimer's disease to death is 2 years, making staff members a more permanent fixture than residents.

Given that the risk of death is elevated in all the elderly residents with or without dementia any GP's patient surviving more than 18–24 months may have to deal with bereavement or loss of a fellow resident. Older patients are often aware of this which may also bias them towards making younger friends. Every reader will know exceptions to this rule, but they are indeed that, happy exceptions.

Daytime activities

The elderly in a home and patients with dementia benefit from enjoyable activity just like any person would in their retirement. Sadly when they are in a home they are restricted by its resources and also the will of management and staff to provide sufficient activity. It is not necessarily the range of activities but sometimes it is the depth or the degree of interest a patient will have in it, which is more important in terms of their overall stimulation and wellbeing. Patients with advanced dementia continue to enjoy, in particular, human conversation, music and dance and visits with children and animals.

The provision of daytime activity may be non-existent in a mutual housing project or warden-controlled accommodation, or it may follow a traditional regime with a visiting external organiser or occupational therapist who gathers residents in a group and encourages them in thoughtful, fun or stimulating activities.

The list of activities which provide stimulation and relief from boredom and loneliness is wide and ranges from singing and simple physical games and exercise through crosswords, poetry, Sudoku and reading newspapers, which also help patients with date and time orientation.

The authors have also seen patients with dementia going out to play golf or swim with a 'sports buddy' although sadly this is relatively rare.

High-cost senior living communities may emphasise the range of activities available but in reality with the advance of senescence, previously active residents need and want fewer of these. Not many older adults maintain their desire to visit the pub or attend concerts or theatres from the time of admission – eventually they may not want to sit in a group watching a magician. The age at which somebody chooses to enter residential care varies widely. A man debilitated by mental illness and wanting to give up living alone in his mid 60s contrasts with the experienced octogenarian clinging fiercely to his independence who suddenly requires 24-hour care in a residential setting in the final weeks of life. For the latter, activity schedules are less important than maintaining contact with relatives or professionals whom the patient has known for a long time.

What would be 'nice to have' as additional inputs?

The following extra therapies have proved to be beneficial for patients with dementia.

- **Regular aromatherapy**: oils such as lavender, lemon balm and sage may produce a calming effect on patients and also promote feelings of wellbeing.
- **Regular reflexology**: can also have calming effects. (Both these treatments also give the patients the opportunity to have calming and comforting interactions with a professional, who can assess them in an unguarded environment. This group will often report their concerns about mood, physical wellbeing and levels of happiness to staff and family members.)
- **A one-on-one carer**: this may be an extra visiting employee who will spend quality time with the patient, rather than a member of staff who is always doing a job. They may eat with the patient to encourage positive eating behaviour, or chat with them while taking them for a walk. As well as the clinical benefits, they also provide another independent assessment on a constant basis.

GPs can tell families that if they object to a specific provision from a home, or wish the patient could have a specific service, they can hire it in, as long as they are prepared to pay for it of course. Families often provide a freelance hairdresser or a physiotherapist. Saying to family members, '*If they like doing it, why don't you hire someone to do it with them?*' gives a powerful message about what the elderly dementia patient may enjoy and applies to nearly every realm of human activity. There is no official comment on the right of provision of sexual services to the very elderly, but arguments in favour of this have been made under the Human Rights Act.

Do patients have to switch homes when they develop dementia?

In an ideal world an elderly patient who is in a home and develops dementia should not have to move. The limiting factors are the depth and intensity of staffing day and night. Small residential homes may only have two lay staff on duty at night, while the largest nursing home may have up to six or eight registered nurses on duty.

Care homes will be approved residential and nursing homes and generally differ according to the number of staff who are trained as nurses. Most residential homes who care for the elderly will have intermittent trained nurse presence, others have a nurse on duty at all times. In the past, registration for management of the elderly mentally ill used to be considered essential to admit patients with dementia for both residential and nursing homes.

On a practical level GPs can advise patients or their families to ask the owner/manager of any care setting: '*What happens if I/they develop dementia?*' The worst answer for most patients although not all, is: '*We don't have anyone with mental health problems here,*' while the best reply is: '*We run a mixed facility with care staff based on site who will begin back-up care as it becomes more necessary. In the future we can arrange for you/them to move to another special unit if you want to have more care.*'

On Golden Pond: living communities

In North America, gated compounds with fantastic infrastructures including services, security and healthcare have been accommodating older adults for decades. These have progressed into towns which are surrounded by countryside and woodland that are aimed at healthy over 65s, but which also contain within them accommodation suitable for dementia patients. By this we mean houses which have structural details suited to patients, like no internal steps or changes in floor patterns which can cause alarm, or which issue temperature warnings when it is too hot or too cold. Healthy partners can live in these houses or very nearby at the same time and services can be adjusted as needed.

The UK is restricted by planning consent and the number of elderly as well as vastly different cultural attitudes and funding. However, a spate of developers have taken old large buildings such as disused boarding schools, army barracks and even former grand country houses to create gated communities or care organisations.

The NICE guidelines of 2006/7 on dementia management advised clinicians, planners and patients to attend to 'lighting, colour schemes, floor coverings, assistive technology, signage, garden design, and the access to and safety of the external environment' when considering residential accommodation. There is a range of practice in these areas, some of which is based on flimsy underlying theory and research. As in much of clinical medicine, trial and error, evolution of shared practice and anecdotal learning are as influential as the more 'scientific' approach to care home design and assistive technology.

The role of warden-controlled accommodation

Warden-controlled accommodation has declined in value both in terms of level of supervision and value for money. They have no role in accommodating patients with dementia. This is because these tend to operate an effective apartheid policy of 'no mental illness here', and their main concern is a wandering patient knocking on a neighbour's door. If a patient is already in a warden-controlled flat and develops dementia they will be managed with heavy input from the GP and social services but will invariably end up in a residential home. Consultant Old Age Psychiatrists are used to being called with: '*Something must be done and the patient must be moved.*'

Exceptions to this are where there is a healthy cohabiting partner or a connected residential home on the same site where the patient with the dementia could be accommodated in the future.

What to advise families about choosing a home

GPs are frequently the first port of call for families seeking advice about suitable care homes. They understand that choosing a home can be extremely daunting and is further complicated by feelings of guilt about 'putting away' a parent or spouse. The following process should help families to make the most appropriate decision.

- Consider the geography: either near the surviving spouse or near the child or other interested relatives, not least because other elderly friends will also move away or die.
- Obtain a list of homes in the area from usual sources including social services care managers and the Alzheimer's Society. Ask neighbours and friends for their experiences and put this into the mix.
- Find out from a GP or specialist if the home needs to be registered for dementia to suit the patient.
- Compile a shortlist if the patient needs nursing home care.
- Drive past the home for an initial external assessment and note ease of access, location, parking, etc.
- Call the homes and arrange a tour. Take account of unanswered telephones, a lack of professionalism by staff and the attitude of managers. Instincts should count strongly in the decision.
- Arrive 10 minutes early for the tour to get a feel for the environment and listen to the staff and patients' interactions.
- If the home smells of urine or residents appear undignified or staff are casually chatting and ignoring them, then have a high index of concern. Clearly some homes will encounter problems sometimes but not all the time.

- Look for wide corridors and doorways, multiple and discreet washing areas, daytime recreation rooms of different sizes and easy access on to secure garden areas. These are all positives.
- Residents' pets should be considered a bonus.
- Chat with other relatives and rather than ask if the patient likes the home it is more useful to ask if their parent is ever in the wrong clothes? This is a classic marker of poor institutional care.

Box 8.1 Activities which stimulate patients with dementia

- Music, simple physical games such as throwing beach balls, word games, crosswords and scrabble type tests
- Newspapers which assist patients in date and time orientation, as well as providing interesting news
- Simple physiotherapy and exercise; singing and dancing
- Some homes provide rarer activities such as poetry sessions and golf buddies

---

Key points

- The most important friendships patients form are with staff in the home, not other residents.
- The level of interest a patient has in a specific activity is more important than the range of activities available in residential homes.
- GPs can help patients decide which type of home will suit them not only now but also in the future.
- Warden-controlled flats have no place in dementia care.
- Families should compile a checklist when selecting a suitable home.
- Pertinent questions like 'is your father ever in the wrong clothes?' inform the decision far better than simply asking if he likes the home.
- A home which permanently smells of urine should raise alarm bells about levels of care.

Chapter 9 **Research, developments and media coverage**

There is a huge amount of research into Alzheimer's disease and dementia underway in a variety of centres around the world. This research spans every aspect of the disease, from genetic predisposition and basic causes through detection techniques, to effective new treatments and possible cures. This research is ongoing and the emphasis of funding and likelihood of breakthroughs will fluctuate with time as it does with any major disease or group of diseases which is as yet not fully understood. This chapter will highlight the key foci of research at the time of writing. The authors are involved in brain research at a leading centre in the UK and will aim to emphasise those areas in which the greatest progress is being made. This should at least arm GPs with the most up-to-date thinking in the key areas, when they are asked about this by patients. However, because of the emerging nature of research, this chapter cannot be taken as a finite guide.

The areas of research which have made the most progress in Alzheimer's disease are genetics and amyloid and tau protein. Currently the latter have yielded a greater amount of research findings. This is partly because the human genome was identified in 1997 but amyloid and tau protein have been known about since 1992. Furthermore amyloid and tau protein are open to more mechanistic and manipulative research while genetic research is far more difficult to conduct and results take longer to achieve. However this position may reverse as time goes on and more results emerge from genetic research.

Genetics

Most cases of Alzheimer's disease are sporadic, and a genetic contribution is difficult to determine exactly, but is presumably polygenic. Several families

How to Manage Dementia in General Practice, First Edition. Nicholas Clarke, Farine Clarke, and Denzil Edwards.
© 2013 John Wiley & Sons Ltd. Published 2013 by John Wiley & Sons, Ltd.

exist whose members exhibit discrete polymorphisms that seem to have a bearing on causation. These include a gene on chromosome 21 for the amyloid precursor gene, and genes on chromosomes 1 and 14, for the presenilin genes (PS1 and PS2). There is also a well established link between a particular polymorphism of the ApoE gene and risk of Alzheimer's disease, though not one specific enough to be useful in genetic counselling. The understanding of genetics has led to therapeutic endeavours aimed at modifying the activity of the products of these genes, and may prove fruitful in the future. Studies in the last 5 years have taken advantage of the very significant reductions in cost of whole genome analysis. These so-called genome-wide association studies (GWAS) have identified genes that make very small contributions to the overall risk of Alzheimer's disease and include genes associated with handling misfolded proteins and inflammation.

There are also known genetic links in some of the rarer dementing illnesses. These include a genetic abnormality on chromosome 9 that is associated with the FTD/MND (fronto-temporal dementia with motor neurone disease) syndrome, and the chromosome 17 abnormality responsible for the FTDP-17 (fronto-temporal dementia with parkinsonism) syndrome.

As yet it is unclear how this may lead to gene-related therapies. However the ability to genetically identify individuals who are certain to develop a 'pure' Alzheimer's disease may assist research into other treatments. Thus the first studies are already underway, in enriched at-risk populations, of some of the disease-altering compounds described later in the chapter.

Neuroimaging

The mainstays of diagnostic imaging remain CT and MRI that help in differential diagnosis of the various forms of dementia by identifying regions of atrophy. There is also some use of single photon emission computerised tomography (SPECT) with radioactive 123-iodide labelled ioflupane (DaTSCAN), particularly to identify Lewy body dementias.

Given that the only way to be certain of the diagnosis of Alzheimer's disease is by examining the brain postmortem for the characteristic hallmarks, amyloid plaques and tau-containing tangles, it has always been considered a considerable advantage to be able to detect these structures *in vivo*.

Neuroimaging of amyloid was originally developed as a response to initial beliefs that the very existence of insoluble beta amyloid plaques in the brain tissue was 'toxic' to nerves. It is now considered more likely that such plaques do indeed reflect the upstream aetiological process of amyloid mismetabolism but in themselves are epiphenomena that are gradations of a pathological process occurring elsewhere in the neuropil (nerve and other brain cell tissue). Development of imaging techniques that visualise tau-containing tangles are much less advanced, but this is receiving increasing attention.

Ligands available for amyloid imaging by positron emission tomography (PET) include:

- 18-F FDDNP – this binds to both tangles and to beta amyloid and is sensitive to change, and is thus a means of tracking disease progression and the effect of treatments;
- 11-C PiB (Pittsburgh Compound B) and 18-F AV45 – the Pittsburgh Compound B is largely the benchmark for two other ligands used in PET scans that bind to beta amyloid. AV45 has been found to have good sensitivity in predicting conversion of mild cognitive impairment to Alzheimer's disease.

Their role as yet seems to be in mapping amyloid deposition in life and correlating with disease and progression, or not. This may enable earlier diagnosis, which, however, is of doubtful utility where there is no treatment.

Palliative treatments

- Cholinomimetic drugs are currently the mainstay of treatment, as described in Chapter 3. However they must be considered a dead end, since they can do no more than increase the function of surviving neurones; the effect is bound to be temporary, as neurones continue to die off.
- Memantine is an NMDA receptor antagonist, licensed for use in moderately severe AD, that diminishes pathological activation of these glutamate receptors. Apart from diminishing pathological glutamatergic activity and tending to normalise brain function, memantine may yet prove to have some disease-modifying effect, since abnormally high levels of glutamate activity activate beta amyloid protein and increase production of abnormal tau protein. For more information regarding this drug see Chapter 3 also.
- Piracetam is used off-licence as a nootropic, or cognitive enhancer, for which use there exists a little supportive literature. The drug's known mechanism of action is as an allosteric modulator of the AMPA receptor, another glutamatergic receptor, but it is far from clear how its cognitive enhancement function derives from this activity. There is little evidence for its efficacy in Alzheimer's disease.
- Other transmitter systems are involved in the disease – noradrenergic, serotonergic and GABA-ergic. Drugs that modify transmission in these systems have been tried, with no consistent evidence of benefit to date.
- Enhancement of circulation by vasodilators, such as hydergine, naftidrofuryl, pentoxifylline, propentofylline, cyclandelate and inositol nicotinate,

has been suggested to be of benefit. Some of these are in clinical use for peripheral vascular disease, but have little evidence in their favour in the treatment of cerebrovascular disease, or for dementia more generally.

Fundamental disease process modifying treatments

In contrast, pharmacological strategies aimed at modifying the disease process of Alzheimer's disease offer some hope, but have not yet proved successful. No new drugs for its treatment have appeared on the market since 2004, despite intensive search for drugs targeting amyloid precursor protein cleavage enzymes and immune therapies against insoluble amyloid plaques. A recent summer of reported drug trial failures, has seen caution grow about the funding risks for pharmaceutical and biotechnology companies involved in this research area.

Beta and gamma secretase inhibitors

This is an upstream approach which tries to prevent pathogenic cleavage of the healthy glycoprotein amyloid precursor protein, as it is inserted in the lipid cell wall as part of normal neuronal cell metabolic activity. Like any such intracellular manipulation it is rife with technological difficulties. One trial of a gamma secretase inhibitor had to be called off because of side effects.

- Semagacestat is a gamma secretase inhibitor that shows good activity in lowering beta amyloid production, but has not been shown to improve cognitive outcome; plans for further trials were recently deferred.
- Beta secretase inhibitors, such as CTS-21166 and MK-8931, have been found to reduce levels of beta amyloid, and even to reverse cognitive decline in experimental animals.

Passive immunotherapy

- Bapineuzumab (Johnson & Johnson, Pfizer) is a monoclonal antibody against beta amyloid, which has been shown by Pittsburgh Compound B PET scans to be effective in clearing beta amyloid. The drug has, however, been shown to lack clinical benefit, particularly in patients with the ApoE4 genotype, though studies are continuing in patients with other genotypes.
- Solanuzemab (Eli Lilly), acting on a similar mechanism, recently also failed to hit the primary end point but there were some positive indicators for more mildly affected patients.
- A promising recent study has shown efficacy of immunoglobulins delivered intravenously (IVIg) in both clearing beta amyloid from the brain

and stabilising cognitive function. (Presented by workers from Weill Cornell Medical College at the Alzheimer's Association International Conference in Vancouver in 2012.)

Increasing interest has been generated in conducting passive immunotherapy clinical trials in populations carrying genetic forms of Alzheimer's disease and in those with established high levels of amyloid in their brains.

Although no likely therapeutic agents have yet been devised, manipulation of RAGE (receptor for advanced glycation end-products) shows some promise in reducing the positive feedback cycle of inflammation, where the products of inflammatory response stimulate further inflammation, and further damage.

Active immunotherapy

Induction of an immune response to insoluble beta amyloid can be achieved by a vaccination based on fragments of amyloid protein. Examples include the following.

- AN-1792 – in 2002, after early promise, a phase II human trial of AN-1792 was discontinued when more than 5% of those receiving the vaccine experienced severe meningoencephalitis (Holmes *et al.* 2008). Postmortem confirmed no difference in neurodegeneration, but did note amyloid plaque clearance, consistent with the original theory. However the worst affected cases also showed T-cell infiltration of the meninges lining the cerebral vasculature.

- This problem was addressed in a modified version of AN-1792, called ACC-001. However this modification has taken the intervening decade, and only now in 2012 have phase II trials begun.

- A recent study from the Karolinska Institute has shown promising results with the vaccine known as CAD106, which stimulates immunity solely to the beta amyloid segment $A\beta_{1-6}$. A three year study has shown no significant adverse effects (Winblad *et al.* 2012).

Science, serendipitous drug effects and dietary supplements

A great variety of treatments have been alleged to be beneficial in delaying the progression of Alzheimer's disease and other dementing illnesses, although none have been proved, and there is only the shakiest evidence for most. Those with more robust but incomplete bench to bedside research findings include the following.

- Antihypertensive drugs – the confounding factors of indication and comorbidity are likely to limit any study into antihypertensives and dementia. Thus despite the known benefits of blood pressure control, the principle mechanisms in dementia remain uncertain. Angiotensin converting enzyme (ACE) inhibitors had previously been shown to be of principal benefit. However more recently a large cohort analysis of elderly US veterans suggested that angiotensin receptor blockers (ARBs) were superior to ACE inhibitors in reducing 4-year dementia incidence risk, by 24% versus 19% (Li *et al.* 2010). A combination of ARB and ACE inhibitor had synergistic benefits, reducing dementia incidence by nearly half. The combination even appeared to slow progress of existing disease, judged by their proxy measure of delay to nursing home placement.

- Statins – there is much indirect preclinical evidence that statins may be of benefit in dementia pathogenesis. Early laboratory findings included reduced secretion of amyloid precursor protein from nerve cells exposed to a statin *in vitro*. Most recently, a study of mice genetically programmed for excess amyloid and memory deficits, an imperfect Alzheimer's disease animal model, showed reversal of cognitive impairment in younger mice on simvastatin, albeit with no effect on amyloid plaques. However systematic retrospective analyses of studies in humans have yet to identify that statins are capable of preventing the onset of dementia or treating the established illness (McGuinness *et al.* 2009, 2010). GPs may sometimes be asked by their patients about media articles that suggest that these drugs actually cause memory impairment. Suffice to say that in March 2012 the US Federal Drug Administration's most recent Drug Safety Review of statins 'did not suggest that cognitive changes associated with statin use are common or lead to clinically significant cognitive decline'. The mean time to resolution of transient cognitive changes is 3 weeks from stopping.
- Brain-derived neurotrophic factor (BDNF) – this has been shown to stimulate regeneration of neurones in animal models of Alzheimer's disease (Nagahara *et al.* 2009).
- PBT2 (an 8-hydroxy quinoline) – this metal-chelating agent is less toxic to humans than the earlier antifungal drugs investigated. Preliminary findings from phase II trials in early Alzheimer's are reported to be promising, but no detailed results are available yet. Metal chelators are thought to act by mechanical reduction of copper and zinc levels in cerebrospinal fluid. This in turn may attenuate the metal–protein interaction implicated in pleated sheet formation of insoluble beta amyloid.
- Oestrogens – as for statins, clinical studies have not borne out the findings of applied laboratory research. The latter has demonstrated that oestrogen improves memory, possibly via oestrogen receptor-mediated cholinergic regulation, acts to interrupt pathological production of amyloid protein and may also act in its role as an antioxidant.

- Vitamin E and other antioxidants – after initial excitement at earlier vitamin studies, a comparison of the cholinesterase inhibitor, donepezil, vitamin E and placebo showed none reduced disease progression from mild cognitive impairment to Alzheimer's disease after 3 years (Petersen *et al.* 2005). A slight delay in progression to Alzheimer's disease in the donepezil group for the first 12 months was not mirrored in the vitamin E or placebo groups. Given that vitamin E has historically been hailed for its powerful antioxidant protective qualities, this study undermined that principle, at least in Alzheimer's disease research
- Non-steroidal anti-inflammatory drugs (NSAIDs) – there have been two decades of research into anti-inflammatory drugs in dementia, with dramatically contradictory findings in multiple studies. These probably served only to highlight the confounding role of patient selection and publication bias in trials. However despite recall bias, studies into lifetime use of NSAIDs do consistently suggest some benefit for patients with the 'higher risk' ApoE4 genotype. This is particularly the case if they consumed larger doses of non-selective older compounds such as ibuprofen and indomethacin for long periods well before the emergence of any dementia phenotype (Imbimbo *et al.* 2010). The concomitant use of anti-ulcer drugs to control adverse gastric effects has obviously assisted later studies. The therapeutic mechanism may be amyloid related, or may be anti-inflammatory via COX 2 pathways for prostaglandin release or reduction in pathological brain microglia activity. One explanation why existing dementia appears to deteriorate with NSAID treatment in some studies, is that these same microglia may also be necessary for beneficial clearance of deposited amyloid.
- Selegiline – this treatment for Parkinson's disease is effective as an antidepressant at higher dose, and with its sister drug, rasagaline, has been researched for its anti-ageing and neurone-protecting effects, perhaps mediated by antioxidant activity.
- Minocycline – also undergoing study in Parkinson's disease, AIDS-related dementia and multiple sclerosis, it has now been approved for a recently started 2-year trial in Alzheimer's disease.
- Phosphatidyl serine – this is reputed to assist in rebuilding or maintaining integrity of neuronal cell membranes.
- Chocolate extracts – there has been a number of flurries of interest about these. A recent randomised controlled study provided moderately good evidence for the efficacy of cocoa flavanols in improving cognitive function in elderly patients with mild cognitive impairment, in performance on the trail-making test and verbal fluency, both aspects of frontal lobe function (Desideri *et al.* 2012).

- Souvenaid (Nutricia) – this dietary additive mixture of choline, uridine and the omega-3 fatty acid DHA, has recently been suggested to improve cognitive function in Alzheimer's disease (Scheltens *et al.* 2012). A suggestion of improved synaptic connectivity is based on a surrogate and non-specific marker, namely EEG activity.

Physical treatments

- Stem cell implants – these have been used with muted success in the treatment of patients with Parkinson's disease and stroke. There is undoubted potential for the use of stem cells in Alzheimer's disease. A number of studies are in the planning stage. Rather than specific anatomical replacement of intra-cerebral neuronal cell types, which is a method filled with hazards and largely unsuccessful, a meta-treatment approach may yield benefits. In this method, the healing capacity of such neurogenic cells would be tested in a drug delivery type model.
- Transcranial magnetic stimulation (TMS) has been tried as a treatment for Alzheimer's disease. In a recent, so far unpublished, study from the Ichilov Medical Centre in Israel, a randomised controlled study of high-frequency TMS showed a significant improvement in ADAS-Cog scores in a small sample of Alzheimer's disease sufferers over an 8-week treatment period.

Adjuvant palliative treatments

A recent evidence-based training initiative across the UK has been termed Focused Intervention Training and Support (FITS). Launched by the Alzheimer's Society, it is designed to bring person-centred care to the fore in a care home setting. The recognition of each patient as an individual highlights the need for an individualised response to any behaviour disturbance. Emphasis is placed on getting a better understanding of individual residents, and particularly teaching staff to understand and allow for their client's personality. Aspects of their personal history and achievements, work skills and hobbies are central to the planning of any day-to-day activity plan, and also how carers intervene when their client is stressed.

Over a period of 9 months, a multi-care home study of FITS showed that antipsychotic drug consumption nearly halved, with no deterioration in measures of behaviour. In contrast clients were described as more engaged and generally thriving.

Other recognised psychological strategies that are at least partially effective include:

- behavioural modification techniques with positive reinforcement of desirable behaviours and extinction of undesirable behaviours;
- skills practice;
- graded assistance;
- cognitive stimulation therapy.

Assistive technology

The Alzheimer's Society website has a good guide to what is already available in the way of devices to help preserve sufferers' safety and to improve their quality of life – see http://www.alzheimers.org.uk/site/scripts/documents_info.php?documentID=109.

Areas in development, likely to bear fruit in the not-too-distant future, include the use of automatic cameras that take pictures at crucial moments throughout the day, which can be reviewed later to reinforce the memory of what one has done. Also, tracking technology can be used for walkers in unpopulated areas to assist patients who are 'lost'.

Ethical and social problems associated with research into Alzheimer's disease

- Insurance risk – the authors have already seen problems with prediction of brain illness in relation to insurance, akin to the notorious example of human immunodeficiency virus (HIV) infection. There is a fundamental tension between the wishes of insurance companies to tailor their premiums to actual risk, and the rights of the individual to privacy, and in the case of HIV it has required legislation to protect the latter. However such legislation does not yet exist to protect those at risk of foreseeable dementia. In the case of Huntington's disease, now that genetic analysis makes it possible to predict a person's risk with certainty, people are under pressure to allow themselves to be tested before being allowed to take out life insurance. A positive result inevitably results in their being turned down, but, in addition, the person concerned may not wish to know their future. Similar problems will arise, on a far larger scale, given the frequency of Alzheimer's disease, when and if tests become available to predict more precisely the risks of developing the disease. This occurs already to some extent in those unfortunate enough to be at risk of developing one of the familial forms of Alzheimer's disease.
- Consent to participate in trials – the bar has risen for demonstration of capacity and best interest in dementia studies, in order to comply with the

research publishing demands of the Helsinki Accord and local ethics boards. Earlier recruitment can help but there will still be problems with enrolling subjects into any advanced dementia treatment trial that has significant risk of incomprehension, discomfort or loss of dignity. As a result cerebrospinal fluid sampling has all but been extinguished from UK and US research protocols, with likely disadvantage to future neurochemistry research. Of the European countries only the Scandinavian patient seems to expect lumbar puncture as a normal part of investigation. The authors also have experience of a patient's wishes to donate their brain after death being outweighed by their family's concern that all brain tissue be eventually returned. This was as a result of the Alder Hey Children's Hospital pathology scandal. Such a stricture obviously could not be complied with, as specimens are subdivided, processed, analysed and safely discarded many times over in any neuroscience laboratory. GPs are in an excellent position to talk through their patient's hopes and fears about research, and perhaps to avoid misunderstandings that can only inhibit further discoveries.

Ultimate hopes for reducing the suffering and costs due to dementia must lie in the elucidation of the causes of the dementing illnesses, and the development of treatments or, better still, preventative measures. There is no reasonable prospect of such research bearing fruit in time to reduce the expected increase in the national burden of dementia over the next few decades. There is, therefore, a clear need for more research, not only into the causes and treatment of dementia, but into ways of diminishing and mitigating this burden. Aggravating this task is that a large proportion of people suffering from dementia are not yet recognised – below 30% in some English counties from Alzheimer's Society findings. There are several ways in which future governments may react to the problem, and most are likely to be by fiat; based on various political theories, unproven and unsupported by research. It is up to those with expertise to do what can be done to influence government as far as possible to act in rational ways. Much of this influence naturally will come from experts appointed by the government itself, such as the National Clinical Director for Dementia. Updated advice from their office is available at www.dementia.dh.gov.uk.

References

Desideri, G., Kwik-Uribe, C., Grassi, D. *et al.* (2012) Benefits in cognitive function, blood pressure, and insulin resistance through cocoa flavanol consumption in elderly subjects with mild cognitive impairment: the Cocoa, Cognition, and Aging (CoCoA) study. *Hypertension*, **60(3)**, 794–801.

Holmes, C., Boche, D., Wilkinson, D. *et al.* (2008) Long-term effects of Abeta42 immunisation in Alzheimer's disease: follow-up of a randomised, placebo-controlled phase I trial. *Lancet*, **372(9634)**, 180–182.

Imbimbo B.P., Solfrizzi, V. & Panza, F. (2010) Are NSAIDs useful to treat Alzheimer's disease or mild cognitive impairment? *Frontiers in Aging Neuroscience*, **2**, 19.

Li, N.C., Lee, A., Whitmer, R.A. *et al.* (2010) Use of angiotensin receptor blockers and risk of dementia in a predominantly male population: prospective cohort analysis. *BMJ*, **340**, b5465.

McGuinness, B., Craig, D., Bullock, R. & Passmore, P. (2009) Statins for the prevention of dementia. *Cochrane Database of Systematic Reviews* 2009, Issue 2.

McGuinness, B., O'Hare, J., Craig, D. *et al.* (2010) Statins for the treatment of dementia. *Cochrane Database of Systematic Reviews* 2010, Issue 8.

Nagahara, A.H., Merrill, D.A., Coppola, G. *et al.* (2009) Neuroprotective effects of brain-derived neurotrophic factor in rodent and primate models of Alzheimer's disease. *Nature Medicine*, **15**, 331–337.

Petersen, R.C., Thomas, R.G., Grundman, M. *et al.* (2005) Vitamin E and donepezil for the treatment of mild cognitive impairment. *New England Journal of Medicine*, **352(23)**, 2379–2388.

Scheltens, P., Twisk, J.W., Blesa, R. *et al.* (2012) Efficacy of Souvenaid in mild Alzheimer's disease: results from a randomized, controlled trial. *Journal of Alzheimer's Disease*, **31(1)**, 225–236.

Winblad, B., Andreasen, N., Minthon, L. *et al.* (2012) Safety, tolerability, and antibody response of active Aβ immunotherapy with CAD106 in patients with Alzheimer's disease: randomised, double-blind, placebo-controlled, first-in-human study. *The Lancet Neurology*, **11(7)**, 597–604.

Chapter 10 **GP questions answered**

What is the quickest and most effective way for me to diagnose dementia in my surgery in 10 minutes?

If someone complains that they have a memory problem they are probably right. Slippage in personal history and biographical details, as opposed to mistakes in the history of the presenting complaint, are a sensitive indicator of long-term memory change. An example would be not remembering the last job the patient did before they retired, or a family event such as the arrival of a grandchild. Using their considerable personal knowledge of the patient, GPs are ideally placed to pick up these 'gaps' as they will know that the patient knew this information before.

Useful further questions which will help to make an accurate diagnoses include:

- *How old were you when you got married?*
- *What year did you get married?*
- *How old was your wife or husband when you got married?*
- *When is your birthday?*

If a spouse or relative has come with the patient try to see them for a few minutes alone. It is impossible in clinical practice to make the diagnosis of dementia at a meaningful early stage without discussion with a relative or person who knows the patient well. They will often describe insidious and progressive deterioration in practical matters at home. These include putting utensils in the wrong drawer when emptying the dishwasher or putting larder ingredients in the fridge. They may also say that the patient becomes more easily disorientated in strange places such as a hotel on holiday.

How to Manage Dementia in General Practice, First Edition. Nicholas Clarke, Farine Clarke, and Denzil Edwards.
© 2013 John Wiley & Sons Ltd. Published 2013 by John Wiley & Sons, Ltd.

The above history and initial testing together will point strongly towards an incipient memory disorder. Having established this, you can then refine the diagnosis with further testing and decide on longer-term management. You can also begin to involve other team members in the care of the patient and their family.

Some GPs may use the GPCOG to help to validate the diagnosis.

What is the first drug of choice I should use when treating a patient with dementia?

In the UK the vast majority of patients with dementia are treated with donepezil (Aricept, Pfizer Eisai). Other drugs commonly used are galantamine (Reminyl, Shire) and rivastigmine (Exelon, Novartis). Prescribing practices may change as drugs come off patent. All these drugs act to block the effect of acetylcholinesterase at the synaptic cleft. However the drug of choice will also depend on the type of dementia from which the patient is suffering, the stage of the disease and on whether or not they have any other precipitating or concurrent conditions, in particular cardiovascular disease.

The initial treatments do not always work in all patients and it is sometimes worth changing within the same group or to memantine (Ebixa). Occasionally off-licence prescribing is necessary for some patients and for this reason GPs may find it helpful to refer to a specialist clinic for drug therapy advice.

What exactly is a memory clinic?

A memory clinic is not a physical clinic like a dermatology out-patient clinic, but encompasses a group of specialists who work together to assess a patient who has been referred, usually by a GP, with memory problems. There is often a system for allocating each new referral to a member of the multidisciplinary team. This means the initial contact may take place in the patient's home or in out-patients by either an Old Age Psychiatrist or another member of the team. As well as assessing the patient, the collateral history will also be taken from a family member or carer at this stage. A second assessment may then take place with a medical member of the team, sometimes on the same day, at a clinic. At this appointment, a physical examination, review of the medical history and any outstanding tests such as the B_{12}, folate, TPHA blood tests, ECG, brain CT or brain MRI will be organised. A variety of cognitive tests will be undertaken as well as the possible consultation with a neuropsychologist who may conduct psychometric tests. At a group team meeting, which is usually overseen by the Old Age Psychiatrist, all the information on the patient will then be collated and a management plan agreed.

How do I access the Admiral Nurses?

Admiral Nurses are senior mental health nurses who specialise in dementia and who have been appointed by the charity, Dementia UK, to work in this role. They provide care, support and advice to the carers and family of those with dementia. Admiral Nurses perform an important and wide-ranging role and can be particularly useful in carer crisis situations, including exhaustion and depression and carer conflict, either with the patient, other family members or professionals.

They also help in management where the patient has dual pathology and in early-onset dementia where family carers may be younger adults or even teenage children. Admiral Nurses keep independent records and their education and clinical supervision are run by the charity itself at regional centres. They are usually employed by the NHS and attached to the local Mental Health Services for Older People team although initially partly or wholly funded by the charity. Sadly Admiral Nurses are not available throughout the UK but hopefully their reach will spread with time, as it did with Macmillan Nurses over the last decades. GPs and the general public can access them directly, and check availability through Admiral Nursing Direct on 0845 257 9406 (www.dementiauk.org).

Whom should I involve to help manage a patient with dementia who lives at home with an elderly spouse?

To a degree this depends on the physical and mental health of the spouse. Having said that, even a fit, competent and active elderly carer will have a greater chance of becoming unwell at some stage than a younger adult. When this person is also the main carer for the patient with dementia, the impact of their absence will be severe if no one is prepared. Therefore it's advisable to enlist as much help as possible when things are good, in preparation for a time when things may go wrong, albeit briefly. Essentially this means having a care plan in place for both the patient and their spouse, so that, should, for example, the spouse end up in hospital, the patient will be covered. Ideally all the services for the patient and their carer including the community mental health team, district nurses, Admiral Nurses and social services will communicate with each other about both parties. In particular any deterioration in the carer's health should be communicated to the mental health team so that they are aware of a potential breakdown in care and make appropriate provisions for the patient. It is worth encouraging patients to start to explore day centres early on, even if they have no intention of going. Some familiarity with these may help patients when the situation becomes stressful later on in the disease.

My patient's children, who are in their 30s, have asked me if dementia is inherited; what should I tell them?

The first thing to say is that inheritance in dementia is extremely rare and as yet the only certain risk factors for sporadic late-onset Alzheimer's disease remain age and a history of brain injury.

All inherited pedigrees identified to date occur at an early age, that is, below aged 60, and this inherited type group represents far less than even 1% of all dementias. This means that if their parent contracted the disease in old age the risk of inheritance, as we know it currently, is non-existent.

For those wishing to understand the situation better, it is worth knowing that very few family dementia pedigrees worldwide have been identified where there is excess brain amyloid protein production or an abnormality in the enzyme presenilin that cleaves amyloid. The resultant deposition of vast amounts of insoluble amyloid in brain tissue is associated with early onset of Alzheimer's disease.

Brain diseases associated with 'pure' tauopathies include a large minority of fronto-temporal lobe dementia as well as some Parkinson's disease, progressive supranuclear palsy and Alzheimer's disease cases. There are only eight pedigrees of inherited tauopathy recorded in northwest England, Australia and Philadelphia and all are thought to be connected to a family which emigrated from Caernarfon, North Wales during the Industrial Revolution. The original gene divergence may have occurred more than 20 generations ago and these families show chromosome 17 abnormalities affecting tau microtubule binding in their nerve cells.

Unlike Alzheimer's disease, the majority of tauopathies, including 40% of fronto-temporal lobe dementia, are due to sporadic genetic abnormalities of either that same chromosome 17, or of chromosome 9. Variable numbers of pathological repeat sequences on the offending chromosome cause diseases of variable pattern and severity, and often with only partial abnormal gene penetrance. This may create an inconsistent 'patchwork quilt' effect of incidence and disease severity across multiple generations. Interestingly at least half of all fronto-temporal lobe dementia cases will report a family member affected by the same disease.

Sporadic Alzheimer's disease and sporadic vascular dementia seem to have little genetic contribution, with only one deterministic gene for apolipoprotein E (ApoE) identified, and its role is not understood. Of the three different ApoE allele types known (E2 E3 and E4) homozygote 'double' E4 allele holders are most likely to be in a diseased group in elderly patient cohorts, but with immeasurable risk. There are one or two pedigrees of CADASIL (cerebral autosomal dominant angiopathy with subcortical infarcts and leukoencephalopathy) gene abnormality causing vascular dementia, and of cerebral amyloid angiopathy causing brittle cerebral microvasculature that may leak or rupture.

The exception is Down's syndrome where such amyloid overproduction is near certain, and early Alzheimer's disease consequently always a risk.

My previously calm patient with dementia who lives in a care home is becoming disturbed and not settling. Can I start an antipsychotic drug and if so which one and when?

This is an increasingly common management issue for GPs. To answer the last part of the question first: there is probably more time than one thinks. A crisis in dementia is akin to what used to be called a 'rumbling appendix' many years ago, and it is worth attempting one or two solutions over a 5-day period. This will have one of three outcomes: benefit, stasis or deterioration. The latter two may warrant relatively urgent referral to specialist services for assessment in the home or in A & E, similar to a surgical referral. For a rumbling community crisis, it is worth seeing the patient quickly to exclude obvious pain, delusions or causes of psychological distress, including abuse or neglect. Having excluded any of these, GPs may then find it useful to then use the following treatments for 1 week and then review:

- low-dose short-acting benzodiazepines such as lorazepam 0.5–1 mg PRN BD–TDS;
- a low-dose, non-sedative anxiolytic, such as pregabalin (Lyrica, Pfizer), 25 mg, PRN BD–TDS;
- a hypnotic if sleep deprivation is aggravating the problem, such as zopiclone (Zimovane, Sanofi-Aventis) 3.75–7.5 mg nocte;
- a low-dose mood stabiliser, such as sodium valproate delayed release 100–200 mg BD.

An antipsychotic may be applicable if the GP is sure of the origin of the problem. That is either it is self-generating or psychological, or medication has been started for a treatable cause such as pain. A suitable first-choice treatment is quetiapine 25 mg OD or BD, reviewed after 3 days and increasing to a maximum palliative dose of 50 mg BD. As always, be aware of QT interval extension in patients vulnerable to heart block.

What is the significance of alcohol in patients with dementia?

It is worth thinking about alcohol and dementia in three ways.

The effect of even low-dose alcohol on the dementia patient's already impaired brain

This is the most common and increasing problem. The key factor is that patients with even mild dementia who enjoy one to two glasses of wine will experience a dimensional increase of the effect. Moreover should the patient forget they have had a drink and drink more this will be akin to overdosing on a drug to which they are already sensitive. Families understand the concept when explained in the following way: '*Giving alcohol to a normal brain is fine but giving it to a brain which has holes in it, is like throwing petrol on to fire.*'

Practical ways of managing the problem include advising patients to stop drinking spirits and change to a glass of red wine a day, or advising families to add tea to sherry, to water down wine, or to provide low-alcohol beer or wine.

The possible causal effect of alcohol in dementia

Alcohol-related dementia is a disputed phenomenon. Two or three decades of elevated consumption may have a directly toxic effect on brain tissue or an indirect cardiovascular effect which raises the risk of mixed vascular/ Alzheimer's dementia, as well as many other somatic illnesses.

Other physical or mental diseases present due to alcohol but which also cause confusion and how they should be managed

All the following will cause confusion and require urgent medical attention before focusing on whether there is any underlying dementia. The most commonly seen is a withdrawal crisis which requires detoxification. More rarely, delirium tremens occurs with disturbed concentration and cognitive performance, accompanied by gross hallucinations. This has a high risk of mortality and requires urgent medical inpatient care. Rarer still is Wernicke–Korsakoff's encephalopathy with its accompanying memory disturbance, gait abnormality and confabulation, which also requires emergency treatment including parenteral thiamine.

My 76-year-old patient complains that he has memory problems but I find him to be very bright and able, and can't find anything significant. What should I do?

As already stated, if a patient, or someone close to them, complains that they have a memory problem then they are probably right. Paradoxically those with high ability and high insight may be identifying early disease and because of their above average capabilities this is less obvious to observers.

Assuming you have conducted these basic tests to reach these conclusions about his residual abilities, you have three choices to discuss with the patient:

- agree to reassess the situation after 6 months, which minimises the inconvenience to his life but increases the risks of failed early detection;
- refer to memory clinic or specialist Old Age Psychiatrist for a global assessment;
- refer directly to a neuropsychologist for psychometric testing – such a specialist is unlikely to be available locally but they may be through a university teaching hospital.

An insurance company has asked me if my 65-year-old patient with mild memory loss has dementia, what should I say?

This request needs to be handled with care. Currently insurers tend to focus on the risks of cardiovascular disease and other actuarially established conditions, but they may increasingly try to assess the risk of a patient developing dementia. Because of this, all doctors need to exercise caution to not unwittingly invalidate a patient's insurance.

It is extremely difficult to translate the depth and extent of any cognitive impairment let alone the aetiology of the memory loss, for an insurance company. If both the insurers and the patient insist on an assessment then it is probably wise to refer for a specialist opinion, although they too will exercise caution in the type of information they will divulge.

It is unwise to simply forward exchanges between the GP and specialist directly to the insurance company without any accompanying interpretation.

Very rarely, we have seen patients in this age group who are under commercial pressure when they sell their company to a purchaser who wishes them to remain for a few years and needs to know about their medium-term health.

How do I know if my 80-year-old patient has dementia or depression?

Some of the symptoms of depression can mimic those of dementia in the elderly making the diagnosis less straightforward. A simple clue is that any somatic or psychological complaint which is worse on waking and gradually improves through the day until the patient feels relief by the evening, but which starts again the next morning, is more likely to be depression. A typical case is a patient with back pain which is worse on waking and recovers through the day, whose symptoms improve with the antidepressant citalopram.

Diurnal mood variation in depression is almost universally in the morning in older adults. This contrasts with some younger adults who oversleep in the morning and experience distress in the afternoon or early evening. Similarly the bereaved may experience lonely grief in the evening or at bedtime. If any symptoms or behaviour get worse towards late afternoon or the end of the day as if the brain is 'running out of petrol' suspect organic brain disease. Relatives may describe the patient as confused, upset, worried or unable to settle during the evening. This is known as 'sundowning syndrome'.

It is common for dementia and depression to coexist in older adults. Rather surprisingly, this is not because they have insight into the fact that 'there is something wrong with me'. It is worth using a good-quality questionnaire, such as the Beck's depression inventory or the Hamilton Rating Scale for Depression (the HAM-D) to aid the diagnosis. It is also worth asking patients if they have lost their joy in life, including their pleasures or appetite. Anhedonia is a core differentiating factor for depression in old age and this differs from symptoms of tearfulness and suicidality which may also occur in other circumstances.

Can I stop a relative selling my patient's house if it is not in their interest?

Fortunately this question does not arise too often. However an increasing proportion of the very elderly, namely those aged over 90, live in valuable property which was purchased and paid for nearly half a century ago. This, together with the vagaries of the economy which affect younger family members, means financial abuse must be considered in some circumstances. GPs with their interaction with the whole family are in a position to detect this before anyone else. The essential component of any decision is capacity, which is dealt with in detail in Chapter 7. The patient is always assumed to have capacity until otherwise demonstrated. This is formalised in the Mental Capacity Act. If a patient knows what their illness or disability is, why it means they must live in a residential home and how it is to be paid for, then they are in the position to make the decision 'yes' or 'no'. They must also be able to understand any advice on the matter, draw conclusions from that knowledge and advice, and remember these conclusions. This applies for at least the duration of the discussion but ideally should remain over the entire period of planning for their move. The patient must also be able to communicate their decision. This means they must not be so deaf, subdued or dysphasic that they cannot demonstrate their wishes. The elderly are also allowed to make foolish decisions just like anyone else. If a GP has any suspicions about financial abuse then they are ideally placed to make an immediate referral to social services, and they should be taken seriously.

Recommended further reading

Books

Ames, D., Burns, A. & O'Brien, J. (eds) (2010) *Dementia*, 4ᵗʰ edition. Hodder Arnold. ISBN 13 978-0-340987-27-8.

Berne, E. (1964). *Games People Play*. Ballantine Books. ISBN 978-0-345-41003-0.

The British Medical Association and the Law Society. General Editor: Penny Letts. (2009) *Assessment of Mental Capacity: A Practical Guide for Doctors and Lawyers*, 3ʳᵈ edition. BMJ Books Ltd. ISBN 978-1-85-328778-7.

David, A., Fleminger, S., Kopelman, M., Lovestone, S. & Mellers, J. (eds) (2009) *Lishman's Organic Psychiatry: A Textbook of Neuropsychiatry*. Wiley-Blackwell. ISBN: 9781405118606.

Hodges, J.R. (2007) *Cognitive Assessment for Clinicians*, 3rd edition. Oxford University Press. ISBN: 978-0-19-262976-0.

Hughes, J.C. (2011) *Alzheimer's and other Dementias*. Oxford University Press. ISBN 978-0-19-959655-3.

Kitwood, T. (1997) *Dementia Reconsidered: The Person Comes First*. Open University Press. ISBN 0-335-19855-4.

Maden, A. & Spencer-Lane, T. (2010) *Essential Mental Health Law: A Guide to the Revised Mental Health Act and the Mental Capacity Act 2005*. Hammersmith Press. ISBN 978-1-905140-29-9.

Marshall, M. (2005) *Perspectives on Rehabilitation and Dementia*. Jessica Kingsley Publishers. ISBN 1-84310-286-2.

Skynner, R. & Cleese, J. (1984) *Families and How to Survive Them*. Mandarin. ISBN 978-0-413-56520-4.

Terrell, M. (2009) *A Practioner's Guide to the Court of Protection*, 3ʳᵈ edition. Tottel Publishing Ltd. ISBN 978-1-84592-244-3.

How to Manage Dementia in General Practice, First Edition. Nicholas Clarke, Farine Clarke, and Denzil Edwards.
© 2013 John Wiley & Sons Ltd. Published 2013 by John Wiley & Sons, Ltd.

Zigmond, T. (2012) *A Clinician's Brief Guide to the Mental Health Act*, 2nd Edition. RCPsych Publications. ISBN 978-1-908020-50-5.

Reports

NICE clinical guideline 42. *Dementia: supporting people with dementia and their carers in health and social care.* Issued: November 2006. Last modified: October 2007.

Banerjee, S. (2009) *The use of antipsychotic medication for people with dementia: time for action.* A report for the Minister of State for Care Services London: Department of Health.

Seminal papers

Ballard, C. & Howard, R. (2006) Neuroleptic drugs in dementia: benefits and harm. *Nature Reviews Neuroscience*, **7(6)**, 492–500.

Banerjee, S., Hellier, J., Dewey, M. *et al.* (2011) Sertraline or mirtazapine for depression in dementia (HTA-SADD): a randomised, multicentre, double-blind placebo-controlled trial. *Lancet*, **378**, 403–411.

Challis, D., von Abendorff, R., Brown, P. *et al.* (2002) Care management, dementia care and specialist mental health services: an evaluation. *International Journal of Geriatric Psychiatry*, **17**, 315–325.

Cohen-Mansfield, J. (2001) Nonpharmacologic interventions for inappropriate behaviors in dementia: a review, summary, and critique. *American Journal of Geriatric Psychiatry*, **9(4)**, 361–381.

Collighan, G., Macdonald, A., Herzberg, J. *et al.* (1993) An evaluation of the multidisciplinary approach to psychiatric diagnosis in elderly people. *British Medical Journal*, **306(6881)**, 821–824.

Cooper, C., Manela, M., Katona, C. & Livingston, G. (2008) Screening for elder abuse in dementia in the LASER-AD study: prevalence, correlates and validation of instruments. *International Journal of Geriatric Psychiatry*, **23(3)**, 283–288.

Corbett, A., Pickett, J., Burns, A. *et al.* (2012) Drug repositioning for Alzheimer's disease. *Nature Reviews in Drug Discovery*, **11(11)**, 833–846.

Cummings, J.L. & Benson, D.F. (1984) Subcortical dementia: review of an emerging concept. *Archives of Neurology*, **41(8)**, 874–879.

Francis, P.T., Palmer, A.M., Snape, M. & Wilcock, G.F. (1999) The cholinergic hypothesis of Alzheimer's disease: a review of progress. *Journal of Neurology Neurosurgery and Psychiatry*, **66**, 137–147.

Gauthier, S., Cummings, J., Ballard, C. *et al.* (2010) Management of behavioural problems in Alzheimer's disease (Review article). *International Psychogeriatrics*, **22**, 346–372.

Gauthier, S., Lopez, O.L., Waldemar, G. *et al.* (2010) Effects of donepezil on activities of daily living: integrated analysis of patient data from studies in mild, moderate and severe Alzheimer's disease. *International Psychogeriatrics*, **22**, 973–983.

Hoe, J., Katona, C., Orrell, M. & Livingston, G. (2007) Quality of life in dementia: care recipient and caregiver perceptions of quality of life in dementia: the LASER-AD study. *International Journal of Geriatric Psychiatry*, **22(10)**, 1031–1036.

Howard, R., McShane, R., Lindesay, J. *et al.* (2012) Donepezil and memantine for moderate-to-severe Alzheimer's disease. *New England Journal of Medicine*, **366(10)**, 893–903.

Karpman, S.B. (1968) Fairy tales and script drama analysis. *Transactional Analysis Bulletin*, **7(26)**, 39–43.

Krishnan K.R., Taylor, W.D., McQuoid, D.R., *et al.* (2004) Clinical characteristics of magnetic resonance imaging-defined subcortical ischemic depression. *Biological Psychiatry*, **55(4)**, 390–397.

The Lund and Manchester Groups (1994) Clinical and neuropathological criteria for frontotemporal dementia (Consensus statement). *Journal of Neurology, Neurosurgery, and Psychiatry*, **57**, 416–418.

McKeith, I.G., Galasko, D., Kosaka, K. *et al.* (1996) Consensus guidelines for the clinical and pathologic diagnosis of dementia with Lewy bodies (DLB). Report of the consortium on DLB international workshop. *Neurology*, **47**, 1113–1124 (updated 2006).

Orrell, M., Woods, B. & Spector, A. (2012) Should we use individual cognitive stimulation therapy to improve cognitive function in people with dementia? *British Medical Journal*, **344**, e633.

Petersen, R.C., Doody, R., Kurz, A. *et al.* (2001) Current concepts in mild cognitive impairment. *Archives of Neurology*, **58(12)**, 1985–1992.

Tanzi, R.E. & Bertram, L. (2005) Twenty years of the Alzheimer's disease amyloid hypothesis: a genetic perspective. *Cell*, **120(4)**, 545–555.

Wetterling, T., Kanitz, R.D. & Borgis, K.J. (1996) Comparison of different diagnostic criteria for vascular dementia (ADDTC, DSM-IV, ICD-10, NINDS-AIREN). *Stroke* **27(1)**, 30–36.

Index

Page numbers suffixed with 't' refer to tables.
Page numbers suffixed with 'b' refer to boxes.

How to Manage Dementia in General Practice, First Edition. Nicholas Clarke, Farine Clarke,
and Denzil Edwards.
© 2013 John Wiley & Sons Ltd. Published 2013 by John Wiley & Sons, Ltd.